"Minshew's *Treating Trauma in Trans People* meets a critical need for gender care and trauma care providers: guiding them in trans-affirming trauma-therapy strategies that are grounded in deep understanding of both the impacts of oppression and the healing of therapeutic and community liberatory practices."

Finn Gratton, *LMFT, (they/them), author of* Supporting Transgender Autistic Youth and Adults

"*Treating Trauma in Trans People* is a valuable guide for clinicians tending to the health and well-being of transgender and gender diverse individuals and communities. The focus of this book is liberation, and it moves us in that direction with a combination of concrete, applicable treatment strategies paired with an examination of the structures that contribute to systemic inequality."

Colt St. Amand, *PhD, MD, (he/they), clinical psychologist, family medicine physician, and coeditor of* The Gender Affirmative Model

TREATING TRAUMA IN TRANS PEOPLE

Treating Trauma in Trans People brings together key concepts from both gender-affirming treatment and trauma-focused care, with interventions focused on resolving physiological, intrapsychic, and interpersonal disruptions. Symptoms related to trauma and stress manifest in bodies, psyches, and interpersonal interactions. Gender, too, is impacted by bodies, psyches, and interpersonal interactions. With chapters that focus on each of these domains, this book provides a framework for clinicians eager to provide trauma-informed, gender-inclusive care. The book then broadens the lens to the systemic, acknowledging the limits of individual interventions when located within a larger framework of systemic oppression and asking clinicians to consider liberation and justice as treatment goals.

Reese Minshew (they/them) holds a PhD in clinical psychology from the New School for Social Research and is licensed to practice in California, Illinois, and New York.

TREATING TRAUMA IN TRANS PEOPLE

An Intersectional, Phase-Based Approach

Reese Minshew, PhD

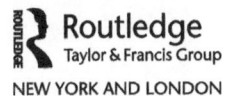

Routledge
Taylor & Francis Group

NEW YORK AND LONDON

Cover image: © Getty Images

First published 2023
by Routledge
605 Third Avenue, New York, NY 10158

and by Routledge
4 Park Square, Milton Park, Abingdon, Oxon, OX14 4RN

Routledge is an imprint of the Taylor & Francis Group, an informa business

Library of Congress Cataloging-in-Publication Data
Names: Minshew, Reese, author.
Title: Treating trauma in trans people: an intersectional, phase-based approach / Reese Minshew.
Description: First edition. | New York, NY: Routledge, 2023. | Includes bibliographical references and index.
Identifiers: LCCN 2022007438 (print) | LCCN 2022007439 (ebook) |
ISBN 9780367681685 (hbk) | ISBN 9780367681678 (pbk) | ISBN 9781003140740 (ebk)
Subjects: LCSH: Transgender people--Mental health. | Psychic trauma—Treatment.
Classification: LCC RC451.4.G39 M56 2023 (print) | LCC RC451.4.G39 (ebook) |
DDC 616.890086/7—dc23/eng/20220624
LC record available at https://lccn.loc.gov/2022007438
LC ebook record available at https://lccn.loc.gov/2022007439

ISBN: 978-0-367-68168-5 (hbk)
ISBN: 978-0-367-68167-8 (pbk)
ISBN: 978-1-003-14074-0 (ebk)

DOI: 10.4324/9781003140740

Typeset in Baskerville
by codeMantra

CONTENTS

ACKNOWLEDGMENTS

My heartfelt thanks to the team at Routledge, and especially Anna Moore, for making this book a reality. Additional thanks to intersectional fat activist and equity consultant Tigress Osborn, who I am also fortunate enough to call my friend. Tigress read this manuscript when it was still in pieces, and contributed greatly to the development and refinement of many of the ideas herein. Thanks, too, to the IBD team at Weill Cornell—I don't always like you, but y'all do keep me ticking.

Many people taught me how to be a scientist over the years. Special thanks to Wendy D'Andrea, Karen Quigley, Andrew Gerber, and the students in the Trauma and Affective Psychophysiology Lab during my time there (notably Adjoa, Jonathan, Ashley, and Steve). You contributed mightily to my scientific imagination and view of myself as a researcher.

Many people also contributed to my development as a clinician. My supervisors and cohorts at The Women's Health Project (notably Lisa Litt and Carole Srinivasan), University of Chicago Student Counseling (notably Anne Brody and John McPherrin), and Center on Halsted (notably Tyler Fortman and Jessica Hudson) were instrumental in shaping my clinical work. I have also benefitted from working with the supervising clinicians and fellows at Chicago Center for Psychoanalysis (notably Peter Reiner and Michelle Sweet). Colt St. Amand and Finn Gratton both facilitate outstanding group consultation spaces—I am indebted to both of them, and to my fellow group members in those space.

More people than I can count have taught me how to be in community. This list is just a beginning, but starts with my large and ever-growing given family: Daisy Reese and Peter Cole; Ānanda Emily Reese, Joe Davis, and Sam and Rowan Reese-Davis; Alex, Katy, Eleanor, Jack, and Abby Reese; Liz and Luke; Hannah, James, and Mateo Barba; James, Ron, Jan, Jason (and family), and Avril (and family) Minshew; Joan Cole and Martin Paley; Susan, Lou, Katie (and family), Lou (and family), and McKenzie (and family) Reese. This work also wouldn't have been possible without chosen family, including Danielle Riley; Rowena Gargalicana; Dani, Jonah, Sam, and Maggie Gabriel; Diane Ehrensaft; Heather Lang, Mary Tregoning, and Mokah Lang-Tregoning; Faith Hillis; Jessica Joseph; Vickie Sliva; Karen Schoonmaker and Miles Whitney; Michelle Ford; Liz McConnell and Ginny Mainville; Gabrielle Meyers; Nancy Serna and Stephen Bohannon; Ebon Craig Therwanger; Molly Lubin and Daniel and Markus Brückenhaus, and so many others.

And deepest gratitude, always, to my clients. Same time next week?

INTRODUCTION

Welcome.

I started writing this book as an attempt to answer, or at least to weigh in on, two questions that have occupied my mind for the past 20 odd years. Of course, they are not the only questions of clinical utility, but they are the questions that have arisen for me time and time again in my private practice, which is explicitly geared toward treating trauma in transgender and gender diverse (TGD) people.

The first question is: how can we best facilitate resilience and recovery in the context of trauma exposure?

While this question has been on my mind for many years, it became clearer and more concrete during my graduate training at the New School for Social Research. There I had the rare opportunity to work with a research advisor, Wendy D'Andrea, who helped me build the tools to ask interesting questions about the physiology of complex trauma. As many clinicians and researchers who focus on trauma recognize, the memory of trauma exposure is not exclusively—or even primarily— a "word" memory. The memory of trauma exposure is, first and foremost, a *body* memory. By extension, then, when we sit down to talk or even think about our experiences with trauma, it is not uncommon for truly remarkable things to happen in our bodies. Our heart rates might spike to 160 beats per minute, or drop to 40 beats, or swing wildly between these two extremes for minutes on end. Our gut motility might dramatically increase leading to stomach cramps and diarrhea, or it might become sluggish and torpid, leading to slow metabolism and a lack of interest in food. Our hormone levels change when we think about trauma. Our perceptions of people and objects around us change, the way we hear, the way we speak, the way we assess threat, all of these are altered when we simply talk about or think about past trauma exposure. Moreover, many survivors are thinking about past trauma *all the time*, which can mean their bodies never get a break. So, assessing psychophysiology in trauma-focused research can yield fascinating and powerfully embodied information about trauma-related symptoms.

In Dr. D'Andrea's Trauma and Psychophysiology Lab, we had the opportunity to both talk with people about traumatic stressors and use lab-based protocols for testing memory, social cognition, and emotional reactivity while simultaneously monitoring our research participants' heart rates, respiratory sinus arrhythmia, skin conductance, and startle reflexes. Sometimes we'd even have the chance to collect data related to brain activity during exposure to traumatic scripts, by playing audio files of personalized recordings while the research participant was in a functional magnetic resonance imaging scanner.

But brains, while fascinating, are merely part of the body, and not even always the most salient part when it comes to trauma. Indeed, sometimes our brains are duped by our bodies into believing that a trauma is happening here and now instead of there and then. As we understand more and more about distributed networks in the brain, I hope we also come to see the brain as a node in the distributed network of the body, which is itself a node in the distributed network of the family, which is itself a node in the distributed network of the neighborhood. One of my frustrations with brain-based research is that it reflects a desire to decontextualize. This book endeavors to make the case that context matters.

DOI: 10.4324/9781003140740-1

Our participants in the lab were so generous with their time and energy, talking as openly as they could about past experiences while struggling to manage the maneuvering of their nervous systems that these conversations elicited. Our bodies will sacrifice our long-term health and well-being for the chance to stay alive in the here-and-now, and our bodies are extremely good at this task. But for trauma survivors, the constant hyperfocus on survival, and the lack of opportunity to ever feel really safe, can lead to a cascade of physiological and psychological effects that, while useful for facilitating short-term survival, endanger long-term well-being.

While an understanding of the impact of trauma on bodies is important, and something we'll spend a lot of time on in this manuscript, it is only one piece of the equation of trauma recovery. How can we best facilitate this recovery, for those trauma survivors who want that kind of facilitation? This is a deceptively simple question, on the face of it. After all, clinicians are highly trained in helping our clients reduce anxiety and reactivity when that is called for, or challenge negative thoughts and understand painful affect when that is called for. Does treating trauma, then, really necessitate a different diagnostic formulation than treating other forms of mental distress? A different treatment approach? Both? Neither? How do we use our increasingly clear understanding of the kinds of changes trauma can elicit in our physiological functioning to afford trauma survivors the opportunity to feel safe in their bodies and alleviate symptoms related to trauma exposure? How do we bend the tools of psychology toward the greatest available liberation from suffering for trauma survivors?

Like most clinical psychologists, I was trained in a tradition of the deficit model of psychology, that centered the question of "what is wrong" with this person rather than "what happened to" this person. But it was in my studies of physiological reactivity that I came to understand the ways in which this position is both problematic and biologically uninformed. Everything that happens in our lives elicits some kind of physiological reaction. These reactions can be difficult to endure, but they are not intrinsically symptoms of something wrong. They are adaptations that have kept our bodies alive in very difficult circumstances. They have engendered our literal survival. Treating an adaptation that helped a client survive as a mere symptom to be "fixed" is doing a fundamental disservice to that person's resilience and adaptability. And, of course, unless there are other strategies online to replace the difficult strategy, simply treating that difficult strategy may call a client's survival into question. When people hold on to a "symptom" as if their lives depended it, maybe they actually do.

While trauma survivors of all genders may have never had the chance to feel safe in their bodies, the bodies of TGD individuals are particularly contested space. TGD people are targeted at multiple levels, from the intrapersonal to the familial to the legislative, because a majority of people in this country believe that TGD bodies are wrong, predatory, or pathological. Which brings us to the second major question of this book: how can clinicians of all genders best facilitate TGD liberation?

Transgender rights advocates know that the TGD inclusion movement has made great gains in the last decade. From bathroom and locker room rights to workplace protections to positive representation in television and movies, the strength of the community has never been more visible. Many TGD people no longer have to choose between living a deeply inauthentic and fractured life or losing everyone they care for. There are advocacy organizations and legal clinics, and more people than ever before who want medical transition are able to access it—sometimes even through an informed consent model that centers TGD people's understanding of our own bodies.

Alongside these positive changes, however, TGD people continue to experience some of the highest rate of exposure to traumatic stress in the United States. TGD people, and especially Black women and transfeminine people, are at greatly increased risk of being subjected to hate crimes ranging from harassment to murder. Our rights are under attack at the state level, and are disappearing at a jaw-dropping speed. TGD people report higher rates of stranger violence and higher rates of intimate partner violence than cisgender comparison groups. And even among TGD people who never experience attack or assault, day-to-day acts of aggression such as familial rejection and employment discrimination mean that gender diverse communities are among the least well-resourced. Indeed, TGD people have some of the lowest employment rates and highest poverty rates in the country, meaning that many of us struggle not only for access to gender-affirming medical treatment but also for access to food and shelter. This becomes a self-reinforcing downward spiral: as discrimination excludes TGD people from the workforce, many turn to the informal economy, which confers a greater risk of exposure to both traumatic stress (such as assault) *and* traumatic experiences (such as arrest) that render access to employment even less feasible. This lack of access to resources, including comprehensive health care, may result in medical trauma, or the trauma of being denied access to the gender-affirming hormone treatment and surgeries that some TGD people want. So TGD people hustle harder, against incredible odds, to sustain ourselves—as our rights are eroded and our bodies are targeted. We have vulnerable bodies in a society that has never been very good at taking care of the vulnerable and has never centered care of the vulnerable as a priority.

If it isn't abundantly clear already, this book talks a lot about bodies, as a way of understanding trauma exposure, a locus for understanding trauma-related symptoms, and a catalyst for recovery from trauma-induced distress. This book centers bodies that have experienced systemic oppression, bodies that have experienced abuse at the hands of family members and intimate partners, bodies that have been assaulted by strangers. This book centers bodies that have been overmedicalized, undermedicalized, and fetishized. This book is a resistance song for bodies that have survived trial-by-fire, and a mourning song for those who didn't survive. This book is about *your* body, whatever your body looks like, feels like, or communicates to the people around you. It is only in bringing our deepest attention to our bodies, whatever kind of body that we have, that we can recover from trauma-related symptoms. But bringing this deep attention can be very painful and scary indeed.

Is navigating the pain and fear worthwhile? This is a real and present question, and frankly, the jury is still out. A host of state-level initiatives targeting TGD children, and the medical providers that work with TGD children, are working their way through those legislatures. 2021 was the deadliest reported year on record for Black transgender women. Globally, the climate crisis is fundamentally just beginning, is already horrifying, and will be the most horrifying the soonest for already-marginalized populations. In these contexts, do I really want to suggest that TGD trauma survivors feel into their bodies? Perhaps, this strategy is premature. Perhaps, TGD people need to be safer, perhaps we all need to be safer, before we can start to be free.

To look at safety in a very narrow way, what would therapeutic safety even look like for TGD trauma survivors? Appropriate clinical care of all trauma survivors is hampered by a relatively low level of clinical training about trauma-related symptomatology. Graduate programs are typically not geared toward formulating clients with a trauma lens, and the vast range of possible responses to traumatic stressors can create confusion and elicit anxiety in treatment providers in every setting and at every level. Even very experienced clinicians can struggle to effectively diagnose and treat the sequelae of traumatic stress and may realize that they struggle with clients who have trauma-related symptom profiles without realizing that trauma exposure is the unifying feature. And if diagnosing and treating the sequelae of traumatic stress is a complicated endeavor, gender diversity may further impact formulation. The clinical care of TGD trauma survivors is hindered by relatively low levels of clinical training related to gender diversity, preexisting judgments about gender diversity, and an antiquated system of psychology that pathologizes difference. As TGD people become more visible, and more gender expansive people disclose their genders to themselves and the people in their lives, clinicians may find that they struggle to keep up with the language and nomenclature of the community, while at the same time seeing gender diversity represented in their client population as never before.

A unique offering of this book is that it draws together two important lenses for conceptualizing treatment. Becoming competent in the treatment of TGD people, but not the treatment of trauma symptomatology, will still leave clinicians feeling lost when they encounter TGD people experiencing the sequelae of traumatic stress. On the other hand, a skilled trauma-focused treatment-provider may jeopardize the therapeutic relationship with a TGD client if that clinician carries unexplored biases about gender diversity or is simply uninformed. A biased or uninformed clinician may even become a source of exposure to trauma for TGD people. And even in non-traumatic situations, TGD people who have experienced trauma are members of at least two vulnerable populations and may feel justifiably leery of being asked to educate their clinicians. We are also exquisitely attuned to lack of safety in relationships, and many of us have already been deeply harmed by people and institutions that were supposed to help us. Thus, TGD people may be very wary of people who give any indication, however small, that they are not to be trusted. This book aims to be a resource for clinicians who want to become conversant with the treatment of trauma-related symptomatology in TGD people and perhaps aren't sure where to start.

This book is also explicit about centering intersectionality. While it is primarily intended to explore issues related to gender diversity within a trauma-informed frame, people of all races, ages, socioeconomic backgrounds, ability statuses, and sexual identities are members of TGD communities. While gender diversity and trauma exposure contribute to marginalization, thus locating TGD trauma survivors as individuals with multiple marginalized identities, trauma exposure and gender identity are only two facets of a given individual's experience of the world. Some TGD people in the United States are white, well-resourced financially, and even Republican (looking at you, Caitlyn Jenner), and their access to opportunity structures will be different than, for instance, the experiences of TGD people in the United States who are Haitian, undocumented, and apolitical. A manuscript that spoke to the experiences of TGD trauma survivors without acknowledging the differences in those experiences across the spectra of intersectional identity would be implicitly erasing the experiences of huge swaths of people. It would also be implicitly centering white, middle-class, abled, heterosexual TGD people. When a trauma-exposed TGD person seeks therapy, that person has the general needs that anyone seeking therapy might have, including some understanding of how their personhood is shaped by systemic influences outside of their control. This person will also have specific needs related to trauma, specific needs related to gender, specific needs related to other aspects of their identity, and specific needs around how these other aspects of identity shape their experiences of trauma and gender. Thus, we as therapists need to have a clear-eyed understanding of these intersections, and a deep acknowledgment of the ways in which our own intersectional identities have shaped our own development. This is not optional or secondary. This is the work.

Because I do believe that this is the work, I strive to be explicit about my identities and my biases throughout this book, sometimes in ways that are uncomfortable for me as a person as well as a clinician. These moments may be uncomfortable for you, too. I have come to think of this as normalizing the discomfort of bringing our full selves to bear on the important work we do. So, I'll disclose some of my positionality here, although I assure you there is more to come. I came to write this book as a TGD person who works primarily with other TGD people, and a trauma clinician who works exclusively with trauma survivors. When I was undergoing graduate training as a semi-closeted genderqueer person, and moving in almost exclusively cisgender or cis-presenting spheres, it was absolutely necessary to compartmentalize the hurt I felt at the stigma and discrimination I experienced. It is very difficult to survive when we try to process through stressful experiences while they are ongoing, especially when we are clawing for a seat at the table of an institution that is innately hostile to our experiences. Because this book is an outcropping of my experiences with anti-trans bias in clinical psychology, and I am a trans clinical psychologist, this book is personal to me and thus may be somewhat more informal in style at some points than a traditional training manual.

Treating Trauma in Trans People starts by introducing framework and terminology related to trauma, gender diversity, and intersectionality. It then goes on to outline the various effects that trauma has on brains and bodies, summarizing theories—and the neuroscience and psychophysiology that supports those theories—that discuss how stress and trauma contribute to dysregulation in our embodiment. The book then outlines the symptomatology of psychopathology associated with this embodied dysregulation and how this contributes to perceptions of unsafe environments and ultimately the perpetuation of that lack of safety. These trauma reactions, ranging from the brain- and body-based through the interpersonal, are grounded in gender inclusion, and considerations for work with TGD people with many different identities are highlighted throughout.

After laying a framework for formulating embodied trauma reactions, *Treating Trauma in Trans People* then moves into an overview of the triphasic model of trauma treatment, which is a model with a great deal of flexibility in its usage. Clinicians who practice from cognitive-behavioral, psychodynamic, somatic, and feminist perspectives will find strategies for adapting their preferred modalities to the treatment of traumatic stress. The phases of safety and stabilization, reprocessing, and integration or reintegration into the community will be discussed from within an intersectional framework that centers TGD experiences.

Finally, *Treating Trauma in Trans People* expands outwards, locating trauma exposure in gender-expansive individuals within the larger questions of what clinicians owe our clients in terms of our abilities to practice radical acceptance and affirmation of all people.

In writing this book, and thinking about and researching the questions posed above, I must acknowledge that I experienced a radicalization in my way of thinking about psychotherapy. Diversity is a biological reality and an evolutionary necessity. One of the greatest strengths of the human species is the behavioral flexibility and physiological adaptability that allow us to function in a wide range of environments—from the clicking hot to the freezing cold, at high and low altitude, thriving on foods as varied as seal meat is from quinoa. Intrapersonal flexibility, interpersonal difference, and community dynamics that allow for both of these are what have allowed our species to survive, adapt, and evolve.

Thus, my hope is that this book is profoundly about radical diversity, radical acceptance, and radical inclusion. In this, I hope we experience an opening of our minds to what it means to have a meaningful life. I am grateful to have had the opportunity to write this book, in part because it has helped me explore—and sometimes explode—my own unexamined ideas about what a life should be. It helped me see the spaces in which I unconsciously center narratives of a particular kind of health or a particular kind of "triumph" over mental illness. Writing this book made me wonder why I ever use the word "disorder" and made me reexamine my ideas about what it means to hear and see things that other people don't hear and see. Writing this book has also made me ashamedly aware of the ways in which the fields of psychology and medicine are innately white supremacist structures that center cisheteronormative and ableist ideologies of what a life "should" look like.

There is tremendous utility in holding an advanced degree in the field of medicine or psychology, however, because we can make these observations from the inside. When we jump through these hoops and obtain the necessary certifications to practice, we have elbowed our way to the table and learned the language of respectability in the meantime. And we can potentially use that skill and expertise to change minds, end harmful practices, and advocate for ourselves and our clients. Thus, this book is intended as a work of advocacy as well as scholarship. The intention is to center narratives that have been overlooked or vilified and raise questions about why psychologists, therapists, and medical providers still have the power to decide who is "really" a particular gender and who is not, who is "really" mentally whole, and who is not. So as writing this book radicalized me, the book itself became a call to action. Every single one of us has the opportunity to work within ourselves to come to a place of true inclusion. Why should any experience—no matter how queer, or Black, or fat, or disabled, or white, or cis—be so outside the range of our acceptance that we can't honor these differences as simply that: difference?

If this book were to succeed beyond my wildest dreams, it would be a roadmap for liberation: *your* liberation. It would be an accessible, well-documented invitation to question the problematic structures that have exercised immense power over our fields since the inception of these fields, and an invitation to imagine new, liberatory practices for you and for your clients. The world is changing. We can change, too, and support each other in meeting the challenges these changes engender.

What are we waiting for? Let's go.

CHAPTER 1

TRANS 101

THE (EVOLVING) LANGUAGE OF GENDER

To be able to talk most effectively about men, women, and the rest of us, it will probably be most helpful to begin with a few terms. In order to avoid any confusion right from the start, I want to lead with a simple truth: transgender women are women, and transgender men are men. Not everyone falls into this binary formulation of gender—a nonbinary genderqueer person is a nonbinary genderqueer person, no matter their genitalia or the clothes they wear. But when I use the word men in this manuscript, I am referring most frequently to transgender men, and occasionally to all men (e.g., including cisgender men). On the occasions in which I talk about cisgender men exclusively, I specify that I mean cisgender men. When I use the word women in this manuscript, I am referring most frequently to transgender women, and occasionally to all women (e.g., including cisgender women). On the occasions in which I talk about cisgender women exclusively, I specify that I mean cisgender women. This is a book by a trans person about TGD people, so I intend that, on these pages, our experiences of gender are the referent experiences. If this elicits discomfort in you, or you find yourself wanting to push back against this formulation, I invite you to take the opportunity to lean into that discomfort and spend time thinking about where it might be coming from for you. Please do not deprive yourself of this time. It will not be safe for TGD people if you attempt to work with us without first resolving this conflict in yourself.

In this manuscript, birth-assigned sex refers to the sex determination, typically based on genital configuration, that someone was given at birth. If someone said, "it's a girl!" when a baby was born, that baby was probably considered an endosex female, and the assumption was that the baby would grow to identify as a girl, pursue activities associated with girls, and over time develop breasts, produce ova, and identify as a woman. If someone said "it's a boy!" when a baby was born, that baby was probably considered an endosex male, with the assumption that that baby would grow to identify as a boy, pursue activities associated with boys, and over time develop facial hair, produce sperm, and identify as a man. So, for many of us, the genitalia we had when we were born (which in some cases was identified and given cultural saliency even before we were born) was implicitly expected to be *the* singular determining factor of our genders and gender roles as we grow from infant to child to adult. And this has big implications for all kinds of day-to-day things, including the clothes we are encouraged to wear (or prohibited from wearing), how we style our hair, how we are encouraged to listen to and speak to others, the sports teams we can be on, the bathrooms we can use, and the expectations projected onto our adult lives.

If you are not familiar with the term endosex, it generally means having genitalia that is either a penis or a vagina. Some people are born with genitalia that does not fit the genital stereotypes of either penis or vagina. The umbrella term for this is intersex, but intersex (as with other sex designations) encompasses a wide range of genital, hormonal, and experiential categories. For instance, a person may be assigned the sex of female at birth due to genital configuration, grow up identifying as a girl, and in adolescence discover that she has androgen insensitivity syndrome. She is an assigned female at birth intersex individual who discovers her intersex identity in adolescence. Many people with this experience grow up to

DOI: 10.4324/9781003140740-2

be cisgender intersex women, but some do not. A person with this experience who grows up to be a man would probably, although not necessarily, be a transgender intersex man. Many people whose intersex identity was evident from birth underwent forced genital surgery as infants, sometimes even without surgeons telling their parents the nature of the surgery or offering other options (and sometimes with knowledge and cooperation of their parents). While some intersex people may find that genital surgery is ultimately medically necessary (for instance perhaps they have strictures that make it difficult to void urine), forced surgery in infancy is a clear violation of bodily autonomy. Depending on how intersex is defined, probably 1–2% of the population is intersex. One commonly repeated statistic is that this is about the same percentage of the population that is innately redheaded. Thus, while being born intersex is less common than being born endosex, it is hardly the rare phenomena that coercive surgeries and secrecy have made it seem over the years. While this manuscript does not focus on intersex people *per se*, I'll reiterate here: intersex women are women, intersex men are men, intersex nonbinary people are nonbinary, and genital surgery that is not actively assented or consented to by the person being operated on is a violation of that person's bodily autonomy.

You may have seen the abbreviations AFAB (assigned female at birth) and AMAB (assigned male at birth) used to indicate birth-assigned sex. Other abbreviations in this realm are DFAB (designated female at birth) and DMAB (designated male at birth) or CAFAB (coercively assigned female at birth) and CAMAB (coercively assigned male at birth). Infants don't have a say in what goes on their birth certificates, so some people prefer to use these acronyms as a reminder that this is an imposed designation, or a coercive assignment, rather than a value-neutral experience. AFAB and AMAB are used throughout this manuscript when it is necessary to talk about sex assigned at birth.

Now, I can hear all of the genderqueer, nonbinary, microboy, and nanogirl trans people that I work with saying, "Hey! Not everyone is *either* a man *or* a woman, you know!" They make a good point, so I want to make sure to speak to some other identities as well. To locate some of these other terms, we will first need to define the gender binary. A binary is any either/or system. The lights are either on or off. And there has been, for quite some time in this country, the belief that people are *either* men *or* women and that these are the only two possible genders. That is the gender binary.

Even in the context of the gender binary, we have understood as a society that sometimes someone was born with a strong identification as a woman in a body with a penis or a strong identification as a man in a body with a vagina. The shorthand for this used to be "born in the wrong body" and was utilized for understanding the experiences of a specific subset of TGD people. This understanding of TGD lives was promulgated over the years by the binary model of gender and the medicalization of what it means to be transgender. For decades, the expectation was that transgender people "convince" a bevy of cisgender medical professionals of the legitimacy of their gender in order to access services, and some of this need to "convince" persists to this day in the form of gender-affirming letter requirements for surgery. But, as it turns out, the "born in the wrong body" experience is the experience of only a part of the TGD community.

While the categories of "women" and "men" do have some utility, and some people of all assigned at birth sexes do indeed fall into these categories, a perspective of gender multiplicity suggests that they can be considered simply two options among many. Other words for gender that you may have encountered are nonbinary, genderqueer, two-spirit, gender fluid, and agender. Two-spirit, genderqueer, nonbinary, gender fluid, and agender people can be of any sex designation and any gender expression—someone doesn't have to "look like" any particular gender to use and identify with these terms. And while there are many more terms than the ones listed here, at the moment these are some of the most common, so I'll go into a bit more detail about them. This is painting in pretty broad strokes, however, so it's always helpful to ask people what being agender or nonbinary means to them instead of basing our understanding of their identities on these categories as broadly defined. People of all genders have different understandings of what gender means, and how our own gender or genders fit into (or transgress) gendered spaces.

Genderqueer and nonbinary people generally identify outside of the gender binary and thus are neither men nor women. Genderqueer is sometimes considered a radical or overtly political label, a way of actively queering the gender discourse by identifying outside of the binary without using the language of the binary in order to stand outside of it. This is a somewhat older term than nonbinary and seemed to grow less common as nonbinary became more widely used but is currently making a comeback as people who may have identified as nonbinary begin to reclaim the genderqueer label.

Nonbinary (sometimes abbreviated as NB or enby) often connotes a similar sense of not being either a man or a woman. While there is sometimes significant overlap between nonbinary and genderqueer identities, some genderqueer people do not identify as NB, and some NB people would not identify as genderqueer. Again, inviting people to share their understanding of their gender (or genders) will be most informative for understanding that person.

Colonizers used an offensive term to represent third or other genders in Indigenous populations of the Americas, and in 1990 the term two-spirit was adopted as a pan-Indigenous, inclusive term for Indigenous people who may have attributes of both men and women or identify in a third-gender Indigenous space (although some third-gender Indigenous people prefer gender identifications that are specific to their languages rather than identifying as two-spirit). Some people who identify as two-spirit also identify as nonbinary or transgender. You will sometimes see two-spirit written as Two Spirit or abbreviated as 2S.

People who are genderfluid tend to have a sense of gender that changes over time, so a genderfluid person may be a man one day and a woman the next, and perhaps another gender or a combination of genders on the third. Some genderfluid people look very different from day-to-day, adopting different clothing and hairstyles as part of their expressions of gender. But some genderfluid people may have the same gender expression all the time or spend years with one gender expression, and what might change is their internal sense of gender. These are all perfectly valid.

People who are agender typically describe not having a gender at all, or sometimes that the concept of gender is simply not relevant to their experiences. Again, agender people can dress or look however they like, so it's important to work toward divesting ourselves of the idea that because someone "looks like" a woman and is wearing a dress that this person is a woman. There is no right or wrong way to perform any gender, and gender is deeply personal. Other people do not get to tell us that we are this or that gender although they may help us understand our own gender or genders more fully.

As conceptualizations of gender grow from the limits of the man/woman binary, new words, terms, and descriptors are being added every day. While the terms demi-, nano-, and micro- were new to me when I attended USPATH in 2017, there are probably several additional terms that have become common parlance in gender-expansive communities that I don't know yet, or that will have grown in popularity in the time between when these words are written and when this book appears. Demi in this context means "mostly," so a demiboy is someone who identifies mostly, but not entirely, as a boy. A nanogirl would be someone who has a small fraction of girl identity, with the rest of that person's gender identity being something other than girl. Other genders that I have encountered sometimes, although in my experience less frequently, are neutrois and eunuch. Neutrois individuals typically consider themselves a neutral gender, and some may wish to have the genitals and secondary sexual characteristics removed. Some identify as agender, while others identify or on the nonbinary spectrum, and still others as exclusively neutrois and not agender or nonbinary. Eunuchs are typically AMAB individuals who identify as sexless and may want to stop their exposure to testosterone (whether via hormonal intervention or orchiectomy).

A DIAGNOSTIC HISTORY OF GENDER

I sat down to write this segment of the book intending to write a brief history of gender as conceived of by the medical community in North America (and before that in Northern Europe). As it turned out, this was impossible—comprehensive information about even this narrow slice of TGD history would have taken the rest of the book, and would have left out some of the most important pieces. For instance, it wouldn't have spoken to the longstanding tradition of TGD Americans, and especially Black, Indigenous, and People of Color (BIPOC) TGD sex workers, as activists, anarchists, and abolitionists. If you are interested in this revolutionary history, and I hope you are, I recommend you start with exploring the work of the Street Transvestite Action Revolutionaries, founded by Marsha P. Johnson and Sylvia Rivera in 1970. You might also take a look at *Transgender History* (Stryker, 2008).

Although I have not personally been around since the dawn of human time (it just feels that way sometimes), it seems likely that endosex trans people, gender fluid people, and multi-gender people probably have and certainly intersex people of all genders have. While it's true that humans have not always understood the contributions of hormones to secondary sexual characteristics, let alone been able to synthesize hormones for stimulating those characteristics in people who want them and don't have them, people have probably changed genders throughout human history. Prior to the understanding of the contributions of hormones to sex characteristics, many cultures had understandings of genders that do not map onto contemporary North American formulations of the concept. Although understandings of gender are changing rapidly in this country, large portions of contemporary society in the United States assert that there are two genders, men and women, and that these are generally predicated on a birth-assigned sex of male or female. But although this *feels* inherently true to many people, and sometimes even so true as to be self-evident, gender has not always been constructed in this way, and it is not currently constructed in this way in many parts of the world.

For a diagnostic history of gender to exist, we must first have a system of diagnosis and then imagine gender as a diagnosable condition, both of which are quite large presuppositions. All of this being said, there are two pieces of diagnostic history that are especially relevant to clinical practice with TGD people today, so I'll use this segment of the book to introduce them. First, in a contemporary, Northern American context, the official diagnostic history of what was then called "transsexualism" begins in 1980, which is when the diagnosis of transsexualism/gender identity disturbance was introduced to the Diagnostic and Statistical Manual, Third Edition (American Psychiatric Association, 1980). The DSM-IV updated the diagnostic category to "gender identity disorder" in 1994, and the DSM-V has replaced this with "gender dysphoria" (the International Classification of Disease, 11th Edition analogue is "gender incongruence"; World Health Organization, 2018), defined in greater detail below.

Second, the diagnostic history of gender in the United States, although in its infancy, has already gone through several rounds of greater inclusion of TGD people and greater exclusion of TGD people. One of the outcomes of some of these battles was the establishment of the Henry Benjamin International Gender Dysphoria Association, which later became the World Professional Organization for Transgender Health (WPATH). WPATH is currently the central organizing body for the treatment of gender dysphoria worldwide, and an educational resource for medical and psychological professionals who work with TGD people. USPATH is the subset of WPATH that incorporates American providers. WPATH meets biannually all over the world (although 2020's conference was located online, like most conferences), and on alternate years the country-based PATHs, including USPATH, hold conferences somewhere in their own country (or online, as it happens). If you are going to work with TGD people, it is helpful to get familiar with WPATH, as this organization puts forth the Standards of Care (SOC) for the treatment of gender incongruence. When clinicians write letters of support for gender-affirming treatment, which remains a requirement for virtually all gender-affirming surgeries and, in some instances, for hormone therapy, we cite the WPATH SOC as our rationale. SOC 7 is the current version, while SOC 8 is under revision and will likely be the current version by the time this book comes out. WPATH is a fairly conservative organization and was initially the province of providers exclusively, which meant that membership was not open to TGD people, as at the time there were no out TGD providers. Many TGD-facing organizations, including some founded by TGD people, have sprung into being in the last 20 years. These tend to be less conservative in approach, but also have less name recognition and influence in the global TGD treatment landscape.

CONTEMPORARY UNDERSTANDINGS OF GENDER EXPANSIVENESS IN THE UNITED STATES

If gender is not solely (or even primarily) the sum of a person's "parts," what is the raw material from which gender is constructed? Diane Ehrensaft, the mental health director for University of California San Francisco's Child and Adolescent Gender Center describes gender as a web, with strands that include chromosomes, hormones, sex characteristics, brain, mind, and culture, among others (Ehrensaft, 2017). Someone might have XY chromosomes, experience an estrogen-forward puberty, have breasts and a penis, work in the construction industry, and be attracted to people of all genders, for instance. None of these things is independently determinative of that person's gender. But all of these intrinsic and extrinsic factors are strands in the individual's gender web.

Another way that clinicians, and especially clinicians who work with children, sometimes talk and think about components of gender is through the illustration of the "Genderbread Person" or the "Gender Unicorn." The Genderbread Person (Killermann, 2016) and the Gender Unicorn (see Ho & Mussap, 2019) invite us to consider sex characteristics (such as genitals), felt sense of identity, gender expression (such as clothing), and sexual and romantic attraction, as components of our genders, and to identify where we fall on these various spectra. Although there are a number of ways of thinking about all of the pieces that go into gender, there is consensus in TGD-affirming communities that gender happens on multiple levels—and some of those levels include various components of our bodies, our felt sense of who we are, how we like to move through the world, and what gets reflected back to us by our loved ones and by society at large.

Because we understand our genders in part through how others perceive us, for some TGD people what is called "blending" (or sometimes "passing" or "going stealth") can be incredibly important. Blending usually means that the individual moves through the world as an apparently cisgender person of their affirmed gender and may choose to disclose or not disclose their TGD identity to others. (I say usually because it can sometimes mean a nonbinary or agender person blending as a transgender person with a binary identity, especially in the context of seeking medical care.) This choice is sometimes made for safety reasons and sometimes made simply because whether or not someone is TGD is fundamentally no-one else's business. That said, there may be all kinds of reasons that someone is disinterested in blending, including personal, political, or physical. And there are a variety of reasons that someone who wants to blend might not be able to. Finally, there might be safety reasons that people choose to blend in some contexts but not others. Many TGD people have complex feelings related to blending, whether they blend or not. Clinicians, whether TGD or not, may also have complex feelings toward blending. But it is helpful to remind ourselves that all of these life choices are valid, and our role is to support others as they make the choices that are right for them. Clinicians should avoid assuming the blending is a goal for their TGD clients, but also recognize that TGD people who do not blend may experience a different kind of psychological load in day-to-day interactions with strangers.

A BRIEF GUIDE TO PRONOUNS AND PAST NAMES

You may be wondering how gender identity and gender expression relate to pronouns, especially as pronouns are some of the most readily shared elements of gender. (By which I mean that it is helpful to know a person's pronouns when talking with or about them, not that it is necessarily easy to share our pronouns.) A pronoun is a word that is used to refer to a noun or noun phrase. I, you, we, he, she, and they are examples of a specific type of pronoun known as subject pronouns. He and she are examples of third-person singular subject pronouns, and for a long time he and she were used as the only third-person singular subject pronouns commonly used in English. As we have moved toward a more gender-expansive society, other third-person singular subject pronouns have been widely adopted and new pronouns have been created. "They" as a singular pronoun was the Merriam-Webster word of the year in 2019, reflecting the widening range of this usage (merriam-webster.com/words-at-play/singular-nonbinary-they). But even prior to the proliferation of usage of the singular "they," most people in the United States had been introduced to they/them/theirs as third-person singular subject pronouns, as these were and are commonly used in situation where a person's gender is unknown (as in, "hey, someone left their gloves on the table"). According to Merriam-Webster, the singular they has been used in this way since at least the 1300s. Currently, there are people of all genders who use they/them/theirs as their pronouns, so now we can use the singular they even when we know a person's gender, if we know that that person's pronouns are they/them/theirs. (As in, "hey, Luz left their gloves on the table.")

Other subject pronouns that you might be less familiar with include ve, per, and zie, although even these options do not capture the full range. Pronouns such as ve and per are neologisms that are intended to move pronouns away from the binary representation of gender presumed by the he/she dichotomy. If you haven't had a lot of exposure to a variety of pronouns you might feel confused about how to use these words or anxious that you're going to get it wrong. While I can't tell you how to use every pronoun perfectly (mostly because I don't know, and also because there will be new ones that I don't know about before you hold this book in your hands) I can tell you pretty definitively that you are going to get it wrong sometimes. The important piece is how you respond to getting it wrong, not being perfect in your pronoun usage. If you find that you consistently struggle to use "they" to refer to one person, for instance, the defensive reaction of "well, the singular they is not grammatically correct" is not appropriate. Nor is flying off the handle when you are corrected, or telling someone how difficult it is to remember pronouns. If you catch yourself using the wrong pronoun, the best response you can have is to simply pause, correct yourself by using the appropriate pronoun, and continue what you were saying. You will probably feel pulled to apologize or explain why you used the incorrect pronoun. While that pull is super common and relatable, it's preferable to work on catching and managing that impulse. When we make an error and then feel pulled to explain, the person who was just aggressed against is being handed the responsibility for managing their own feelings AND the feelings of the person who has just mispronounced them. Sorting through those feelings ourselves, or with a trusted friend, rather than the person we just hurt, will be a better fit for all concerned. A similar reaction is preferred if you don't happen to catch yourself, but rather have the experience of someone else correcting you. A simple "oh, thank you," and then continuing with what you were saying using the correct pronoun, acknowledges the error without trying to justify or explain intent.

If you don't already spend time in LGBTQ+ or TGD spaces, you might not know that asking people's pronouns is a common practice in these spaces and not something to feel shy or self-conscious about. It can help to lead with offering your own pronouns before you ask for someone else's. A simple, "My name is Frankie, I use he/him or per/pers…what are your name and pronouns?" can become second nature with just a bit of practice. That said, if you are going to ask anyone for pronouns, especially during group introductions, please make sure you're asking everyone and not just people who "look like" you should. We really can't tell someone's gender just by looking, and we also can't tell their pronouns without asking.

On that note, it is also helpful to work on getting comfortable being asked your own pronouns. You might initially feel insulted (*can't you tell what my pronouns are?*) or tempted to qualify (*I use she/her, obviously*) or to diffuse your discomfort through the jocular answer of giving pronouns that aren't the ones you use or giving some random nouns as your pronouns. Although it is not uncommon for people to do this as a joke (Chris Cuomo, for instance, at the LGBT Town Hall sponsored by CNN and the Human Rights Campaign), it is a form of "punching down" or using people with less power in society as the punchline of your joke. Please avoid this. If you are asked your pronouns, some appropriate responses are "My pronouns are he/him/his, or anything used with respect," "I use they/them," or "please just use my name."

If you spend time in gender diverse spaces, you will inevitably hear someone else use a pronoun that you believe is incorrect to describe a third party. If you're confident that the third party uses the same pronouns in all contexts, it is completely appropriate (and a helpful piece of allyship) to intervene. Generally, a helpful intervention is along the lines of, "Oh, I think Shaz uses she/her." If you know that she/her might be newer for Shaz, or not the right pronouns in every context, check in with Shaz first and ask if she would like for you to correct people moving forward. And after you've checked in, make sure to support her in the ways she has requested.

Much of this information applies to past names as well, including the name that may be on a person's state-issued identification card, insurance card, or birth certificate, but is not the name that person uses currently. Past names (sometimes also called "dead names" or "birth names") are private information for many TGD people. If you don't know the name that someone used to use, please don't ask—this person will tell you if it becomes necessary or relevant. If you *do* know someone's past name, either because you have seen a form of identification that has that name, or you have known the person since they used that name, it is most helpful to mentally silo this information about them. You should not call someone by their past name unless they have specifically asked you to do so in a particular context (you are interfacing with a health care provider to whom they have not disclosed the name they use, for instance). Nor should you disclose someone's past name to anyone else. (The most common way this happens is when we're are establishing mutual relationships, as in, "You know Sylvia who used to be Ed, right?" There are other ways to establish this information.)

THE ROLE OF THE CLINICIAN IN WORKING WITH TGD PEOPLE

What is called gender dysphoria (DSM-V) or gender incongruence (ICD-11) can be defined as a strong feeling of disconnection between one's gender identity and one's body. Although we as providers may work with TGD people on any number of life concerns, simply being transgender or gender diverse is not a diagnosis, a cause for medical intervention, or a pathology. When TGD people seek services for posttraumatic stress disorder, or depression, or anxiety, we should diagnose them with posttraumatic stress disorder, depression, or anxiety. It is only when someone is experiencing this disconnection between their gender identity and their body that we should diagnose gender dysphoria or gender incongruence. Indeed, there is significant controversy over whether or not gender dysphoria/gender incongruence should be diagnosable conditions, as they simply reflect the diversity of human life. However, at this moment we use a system of diagnosis to obtain appropriate treatment for our clients, and by the logic of this system, gender dysphoria or gender incongruence can be appropriately diagnosed in the pursuit of appropriate interventions.

Because of a longstanding history of pathologization of TGD people in the United States, it is important to recognize that many TGD people never seek medical treatment, whether to manage gender expression or for any other reason. In fact, TGD people are frequently hesitant about seeking needed medical care, dental care, or preventative care, in part because we never know if a treatment provider will be competent to work with TGD people. We have reason to be skeptical—according to the data from the 2015 US Transgender Survey, a third of TGD people who had seen a doctor in the last year reported at least one negative provider experience related to provider transphobia (James et al., 2016). These range from having to educate doctors, nurses, and physician's assistants about gender to experiences of violence, sexual assault, and refusal of treatment from medical personnel. The survey was conducted in 2015, and there was a change in federal administration in 2016 that made it even easier for medical care providers to discriminate against TGD people under the guise of religious liberty. At the time I am editing this manuscript, the federal administration has again changed and is rolling back some of the roll backs of 2016–2020. However, conservative states are stepping into this territory in a major way, as I'll discuss in greater detail in the section about TGD youth. Thus, it is important to remember that most TGD people have the perception that our bodies are not safe, and feel they may be especially unsafe with medical providers. This feeling of being unsafe is not paranoia, but based on both historical data and contemporary experiences.

Some of the ways that TGD people are affirmed in our genders are social transition and medical transition, which might include hormone treatment and/or surgery. Not everyone necessarily wants any or all of these interventions. Some men are very comfortable with their vaginas and breasts, while some women love their flatter chests and penises. People can be TGD without changing their bodies, changing their clothes, or changing their names, although many TGD people choose to change some or all of these things. It is my position (and the position of many people in the field, many TGD people, and many TGD people in the field) that when a person tells you their gender, that is their gender, and we should let go of the toxic culture of asking for "proof." This insistence on proof that we find legible has a great deal of painful fallout and has been the backbone of gatekeeping and denial of services. Let's move toward a system wherein we take people at their word when they tell us who they are. As it turns out, this desired system has a name: the gender affirmative model or the gender-affirming model. For a multidisciplinary overview of this model as pertains to children, see Keo-Meier and Ehrensaft (2018). For an overview as relates to medical care, including primary care, see Deutsch (2016). For a medical view focused on HIV prevention, see Reisner et al. (2016).

SOCIAL TRANSITION

For individuals who *do* want to pursue some form of outward-facing transition, some of the options available to them might include various forms of social transition. Social transition might include changing hair length or style, using a different name and/or different pronouns, and wearing different clothes (or the same clothes but with a different style or different accessories). People with fuller chests who want flatter chests may "bind," flattening their chests using compression garments known as binders, or with a special, skin-friendly tape. People with flatter chests who want fuller chests may wear padded bras to fill out their chests. Some people may use "packers," which create a genital bulge for people who want one (some also allow a user to urinate standing up). Some people "tuck" and use compression underwear, gaffs, or special tape to create a flatter genital region (tape will prevent the user from urinating for the duration of tucking).

As a part of social transition, people may choose to legally change their name and/or their gender marker with the court. For people who want to change their legal name and/or gender marker, there are a number of barriers to access. For one thing, in most places, this change involves publishing your intention to change your name in a newspaper or similar (which carries a cost and can also increase risk for people who are, for instance, escaping domestic violence). Then, one must file an application with the court, which is a barrier for people with lower literacy and also may be a barrier for people who have been involved with the carceral state, including anyone who has outstanding fines or a warrant. Once the application is successfully filed, one is given a court date, which is a fixed date and time during the work week. Going to the court date requires transportation at that particular date and time and thus has potential transportation barriers and financial barriers, especially for hourly workers. Then the document must be sealed and filed with the court. This process generally costs around $300 outright, plus associated costs as mentioned above, and that's just for the name and/or gender marker change with the court. Then there is the cost of time and money associated with getting new documentation from social security (if one has a social security number) and from the state (e.g., a driver's license or state ID), and, for citizens and documented residents who want to travel internationally, from the federal government (e.g., a passport). In some situations, it is helpful to change one's birth certificate as well, which is an additional barrier of paperwork, time, and money. If your gender is not on the gender binary, in many situations, this will also feel like an exercise in futility, as most states only allow the option of "M" or "F" as gender markers. This means that your option might be to go from one wrong gender marker to another wrong gender marker, which is hardly appealing. Moreover, every single one of these interactions leaves the person vulnerable to acts of aggression ranging from microaggression to assault. All of which is to say that many people who use a different name or gender marker than the original do not make these changes with the court system, and instead simply start using a new name and/or pronouns. Thus, there are many reasons why someone might have identification with a picture, name, or gender marker that does not match their current presentation, so this is something to be mindful of when you begin working with a new person who may be considering social transition or in the process of social transition.

MEDICAL TRANSITION: HORMONE REPLACEMENT THERAPY

People who want to change their bodies to better reflect their gender identity sometimes choose hormone replacement therapy or HRT (sometimes called gender-affirming hormone therapy or GAHT). The information about HRT described below will typically be imparted to your clients who seek HRT in greater detail by their hormone prescribers (and many of them will already know this information from online research and community members). But as providers we should be aware of the trajectory of changes someone might notice with HRT. For one thing, HRT can impact mood, especially early on, and it's useful for those of us who work with people on mood-related differences to be aware of this! For another, many people who start HRT are excited to talk about the changes they're noticing in their bodies, and your knowledgeability will help create a safer environment to share this excitement. Additionally, if you have the capacity to prescribe medication, you may choose to prescribe HRT. While this book is not a guide for prescribing or any form of medical intervention, nor should anything in here be construed as medical advice, there are many resources available to you if you do decide to begin offering HRT as a resource to the community, and you would be offering a valuable service option for people who are historically marginalized and underserved. Finally, depending on the state in which you provider clinical care and the age of your clients, you may be asked to write letters of support for hormone therapy. In a letter of support, one generally affirms that the individual seeking hormones or surgery has a clear understanding of the possible risks and benefits, which means that you also need an understanding of the risks and benefits. So I hope this information will be helpful to you, with the caveat that there it is a glancing overview and not comprehensive.

As providers we should also be aware of the barriers to access around HRT, one of the most significant of which is financial. While it is now illegal for many health care insurance plans to have blanket exclusions of coverage for transition-related care, TGD people continue to face discrimination in accessing coverage for HRT and surgery. And while Medicare and Medicaid are required to cover transition-related treatment, TGD people with Medicare and Medicaid also face a variety of obstacles for coverage of transition-related care. This is exacerbated in states that require mental health provider letters of support for initiation of HRT (for instance, an insurance plan may cover the HRT, but not have behavioral health benefits, or there may be no in-network gender-affirming mental health provider in someone's area). This is on top of the non-specific financial difficulties of accessing any kind of health care in the United States—high deductibles, pharmacy plans that don't cover the specific preparation you were prescribed, long waitlists for specialty providers, and plain old lack of coverage. Additionally, many states are currently working to dramatically restrict access to HRT, especially for those under the age of 18.

When people are able to navigate these barriers, and the social barriers they may also be facing, here are some of the effects of HRT that they might expect. For adults who endogenously produce higher testosterone, and do not want the bodily effects of higher testosterone, there are medications that reduce or suppress the amount of testosterone they produce. The most commonly prescribed testosterone suppressant is spironolactone, which was designed as a diuretic and treatment for hypertension, and only incidentally discovered to also be a testosterone suppressant. I want to tag this as an effect because most people notice an increased need to urinate when they start on spironolactone, and bathrooms can be very difficult spaces for TGD people. Talking about feelings related to gender-segregated bathrooms, and safety-planning for bathroom use, is important for all TGD people, and may be especially salient for TGD people starting on spironolactone. Testosterone-producing people may also stop producing testosterone via orchiectomy, described below.

Because adult humans require some sex hormones for bone density and energy, and many people who don't want the effects of testosterone DO want the effects of estrogen, people who use spironolactone to suppress testosterone, and are under the typical age of menopause, often also use estrogen and sometimes progesterone. Sometimes people can achieve blood levels of estrogen that suppress the effects of testosterone without the continued use of spironolactone. This will vary by a person's body, desired effects, and the amount and mode of administration of the estrogen, which can be administered via injection, orally, or transdermally.

The suppression of testosterone and addition of estrogen tends to have several physical and emotional effects. The physical effects are thinning of skin, reduction in sweat, and sometimes a change in the odor of the individual's sweat and urine. Fat distribution and muscle mass change, with fat accumulating more on the hips and thighs and less in the belly, and muscle mass and strength decreasing overall. A person with reduced or suppressed testosterone and added estrogen will typically begin to develop breasts. More recently, the addition of progesterone has been used to increase breast development. Hormone protocols combined with breast pumping have been shown to successfully induce lactation if this is a goal. The growth of body hair and facial hair slow down, although they do not stop altogether. Many people report emotional changes, although this is a variable process and different for everyone. Some people report feeling much happier, as their bodies are changing in ways that affirm their gender. Some report sadness and low energy as their bodies adjust to the effects of decreased testosterone. Sexual function also changes—people with penises who are suppressing testosterone and/or taking estrogen may find that they have changes in their ability to establish or maintain an erection, and some report a change in the size and shape of their genitals as well as a difference in the intensity of orgasm or the time it takes to reach orgasm. On the issue of fertility, in most cases, suppression of testosterone and initiation of estrogen results in non-viable sperm while using this combination of medications. Sometimes, people who stop using these treatments regain the ability to produce viable sperm, but there is a great deal of competing information about the probability of this. Adults who are considering suppressing testosterone and initiating estrogen should talk with a gender-affirming fertility specialist if they would like to have children that are genetically related to them, and all of their providers should be prepared to talk about family planning. Finally, past or current suppression of testosterone and/or addition of estrogen should not be considered a method of birth control.

While many women and feminine-spectrum people who endogenously produce testosterone see a softening of their features and reduction of body and facial hair with the suppression of testosterone and addition of estrogen, there are some effects of a testosterone-forward puberty, such as the squaring of a jaw and protrusion of a brow ridge, that remain the unchanged. By and large, the pitch and timbre of a voice that has "dropped" will also remain the same. For people who have had a testosterone-forward puberty and want a higher voice, voice coaching can be helpful for addressing this form of gender incongruence, and there are also surgical procedures as described below that can reduce the size of the vocal apparatus resulting in a higher-pitched voice. For people with unwanted facial and body hair, electrolysis or laser hair removal can be helpful. Of course, these services are expensive, and sometimes necessitate lengthy recovery. They can also contribute to increased dysphoria or incongruence in the short-term—electrolysis, for instance, requires that a person let their hair grow out a bit prior to treatment, which can be very upsetting for women and feminine-spectrum people with unwanted facial hair. It should also be noted that women and feminine-spectrum people who want inversion vaginoplasty will likely be advised to seek electrolysis or laser hair removal at the donor site for perhaps a year prior to surgery. Even in pursuit of a much-wanted surgery, this is an awkward and uncomfortable process that can aggravate gender incongruence as well as something to consider in the timeline of pursuit of vaginoplasty.

Adults who have had an estrogen-forward puberty, and begin utilizing testosterone as HRT, will also notice a change in the odor of their sweat and/or urine, as well as a thickening of skin, and a redistribution of body fat away from the thighs and hips and toward the belly. They will also generally find it easier to develop muscle and will get stronger faster and with less load-bearing activity. Over time they will notice an increase in body hair and facial hair, although the capacity to grow a beard or mustache may take several years to develop (as with any testosterone-forward puberty). Some people notice thinning hair or balding, depending on genetic predisposition toward baldness. Some people describe emotional changes such as finding it easier to get angry and more difficult to cry, although this is very variable. Most people utilizing testosterone experience vocal changes as their vocal apparatus becomes larger and less mobile, although there are dosing schedules that make voice changes less likely if someone wants to maintain their original voice. Generally, there is a squaring of the jaw and thickening of the brow ridge associated with all testosterone-forward puberties. Almost everyone utilizing testosterone reports an increased sex drive and intensification of orgasm. Many people notice a change in the size and shape of their genitals, and many describe a change in their sexual desire. Some men and masculine-spectrum people using testosterone will experience a cessation of menstruation, although those who don't are sometimes prescribed birth control (generally progesterone-only birth control) for menstrual suppression if desired. Indeed, this may also be helpful for the conventional reason of avoiding pregnancy—while testosterone may impact ability to conceive, it is not a birth control method. One study suggests that a third of pregnancies in men are unplanned, although not all of the men in the study utilized testosterone (Light et al., 2014). Thus, it is important for those of us who work with TGD people to be comfortable talking about the possibility of pregnancy experienced by men and masculine-spectrum people and not to make assumptions about the ways in which men and masculine-spectrum people might be having sex. People who are planning to initiate testosterone, and would also like to have genetically related children, should talk with a gender-affirming fertility specialist about their options. It should be noted that fertility-preservation options for AFAB people (of any gender) are more expensive, more invasive, and less sure than fertility-preservation options for AMAB people (of any gender).

As with estrogen, there are some things that testosterone alone does not do. Although testosterone does contribute to the redistribution of body fat, it does not eliminate (or even significantly reduce) breast tissue that has already developed. Some people using testosterone for gender affirmation will choose top surgery (described below) or other forms of body shaping to address this form of gender incongruence. Testosterone also does not change pelvic structure, so people with a wider pelvis will continue to have wider hips, even with a redistribution of body fat. And, although most people using testosterone will ultimately notice a change in the shape and size of their genitals, this will not enable most to comfortably urinate while standing.

MEDICAL TRANSITION: SURGERIES

Gender-affirming surgeries are life-affirming surgeries. They are, not infrequently, life-saving surgeries. They are also medical procedures that have been created and practiced by cisgender surgeons on TGD bodies. This is becoming less true—as social space and activism have offered some TGD people greater access to opportunity, there are more TGD surgeons. As gender-affirming surgeries have been legalized and recognized as medically warranted for gender incongruence (and also as lucrative procedures), there has been an increased interest in developing surgical techniques to improve outcomes and patient comfort. But cisgender clinicians should always keep in mind the compounded stress of being a TGD person in need of medical support. Judgments from health care providers, even those who work frequently with TGD people, are frequent, and can run the gamut from misgendering by an administrative staff member through to medical malfeasance. When we receive medical attention, and especially surgery, our bodies are at their most vulnerable and we are at our most defenseless. All surgery carries the risk of post-surgical complication, including pain. Post-surgical pain is something to talk about with all of our clients who are seeking surgery, and especially with TGD people who have experienced trauma and stress. The experience of surgery can be a trigger for people who have been physically or sexually maltreated or assaulted, as it combines the experiences of pain and being out of control. Gender-affirming surgeries also frequently incorporate having strangers look at and touch sensitive and private areas of the body, and areas that may be associated with shame, discomfort, and dysphoria.

These are entirely valid concerns that you will hear when your TGD clients are considering surgery. At times, hearing clients express these concerns may elicit the desire in you to "gatekeep" or refuse to write a letter of support for that person's surgery. (For most gender-affirming surgeries to be covered by insurance, or even for most surgeons to consider offering an individual this surgery, the person will need at least one letter of support and sometime two from a mental health professional, and one from a medical professional, so this is not an abstraction.) I want to normalize talking about TGD concerns about surgery, and expand our collective capacity to recognize that ambivalence about surgery and a period of mourning around surgery does not indicate that surgery is the wrong choice or the process should be delayed due to *provider* ambivalence. To help reduce that ambivalence, I'll just briefly bring your attention to the success rates of gender-affirming surgeries. There is a growing misapprehension that a large percentage of TGD people who choose gender-affirming surgeries come to regret these surgeries, which is simply untrue. Gender-affirming surgeries have an exceptionally low rate of expressed regret and worry that an individual might express regret is not a compelling argument for withholding treatment (McQueen, 2017). TGD people who have gender-affirming surgery rarely report major regret, and minor regret (which seems to affect about 5% of people who have gender-affirming surgery) tends to be directed toward post-surgical complications and results rather than the decision to seek a gender-affirming procedure (van de Grift et al., 2018). When people have gender-affirming surgery, their experience of gender incongruence is decreased and typically their quality of life is improved.

While clinician ambivalence is a barrier to gender-affirming surgery, it is far from the being the only obstacle. Financial considerations include all of those described above regarding hormone therapy, plus additional financial barriers in the form of needing time away from work, and a physically and psychologically safe-enough place for recovery. This may include factoring in additional time for recovery if there is a complication, or if a revision is needed.

Another significant barrier to surgical care is anti-fat bias. Many plastic surgeons, who would be the primary providers of non-genital surgery, have body mass index (BMI) limits and will not provide care for individuals outside of these limits. Most surgeons who offer genital surgery also have BMI limits. The BMI is a measure that is rooted in medical racism and especially anti-Black bias (see Strings, 2019). While surgeons have the right to make decisions about who they will and won't serve, the most recent data indicate that BMI is an arbitrary metric for making this decision (Brownstone et al., 2021).

TYPES OF GENDER-AFFIRMING SURGERIES

When people are able to traverse these barriers and opt for gender-affirming surgery, these are some of the surgeries currently available. Top surgery, sometimes called chest masculinization, is a double mastectomy with contouring to remove the breast tissue and create a chest that looks like the chest of someone who has had a testosterone-forward puberty. There are several ways in which this can be achieved depending on the size and shape of the person's chest. Top surgery is typically an outpatient procedure performed by a plastic surgeon. This is by far the most sought-after surgery for men and masculine-spectrum people who have had an estrogen-forward puberty.

Other surgeries for men and masculine-spectrum people include an array of facial surgeries, which may include rhinoplasty, jaw-shaping, and thyroid cartilage enhancement (building up the "Adam's apple"). Other body-based plastic surgeries may include liposuction to shape the flanks and thighs.

Bottom surgery for people born with vaginas or other kinds of genitals and who would like to have a penis typically means either metoidioplasty or phalloplasty. Metoidioplasty, sometimes called a "meta," unhooks the clitoral tissue from the surrounding tissue (most notably a ligament that holds it to the pubic bone), releasing it to its full length, and thus is an option for many people with a clitoral glans. Post-operative size will depend on the individual, and also on if the person is using or has used testosterone for long enough to have genital growth, but a person who obtains a meta will ultimately typically have a neopenis of 1–3 inches. A metoidioplasty can be performed with or without urethral lengthening, and if performed with urethral lengthening, most people who have had the procedure will be able to urinate while standing. Metoidioplasty can be performed with or without associated interventions, which might include testicular implants, vaginectomy, and hysterectomy. It does not diminish sexual or tactile sensitivity, and the tissue is erectile tissue, meaning that the neopenis can become erect without additional surgical intervention.

The other surgical option for people with vaginas and other genitals who would like a penis is called phalloplasty. During phalloplasty, a neopenis is created from skin harvested from the forearm or upper thigh, or sometimes the groin, abdomen, or back muscle. Phalloplasty may require several rounds of surgery depending on the various options and also on complications—two to five rounds of surgery is fairly typical. Because the clitoral glans tissue is left intact near the base of the neopenis, most people who are able to reach orgasm prior to surgery can have an orgasm after surgery as well. However, because the neopenis is constructed from tissue that is not erectile, it typically requires the installation of an erection pump for the person to be able to have an erection. Many people who have had phalloplasty can ultimately urinate while standing, although in some cases strictures or other difficulties with healing inhibit that possibility.

There are also a number of surgeries that women and feminine-spectrum people who had a testosterone-forward puberty might be interested in. Facial feminization surgery is used as an umbrella term for a number of possible facial surgeries and combinations of facial surgeries. These may include brow reduction, rhinoplasty, chin reshaping, and tracheal shave.

Other surgeries that women and feminine-spectrum people who had testosterone-forward puberties might seek are breast augmentation (sometimes also called top surgery), orchiectomy, and vaginoplasty. In most cases, surgeons recommend at least a year of HRT prior to breast augmentation to maximize pre-surgical breast development.

Women and feminine-spectrum people with external testicles sometimes pursue orchiectomy, which is the removal of testicles through a small incision in the scrotum. For women and feminine-spectrum people who endogenously produce testosterone, an orchiectomy (sometimes called an orchi, pronounced or-key) can provide a great deal of relief from gender dysphoria, as the surgery has the same effect as a testosterone blocker such as spironolactone without necessitating medication for the purpose. Some women and feminine-spectrum people who have orchiectomies find that they are able to use less estrogen to maintain desired effects after the procedure, which can help improve orgasm quality and firmness in women and feminine-spectrum people who opt to keep their penises. For those who have penises and want vaginas, orchiectomy is also considered a precursor of vaginoplasty, particularly for those seeking a penile inversion (although in some instances these are performed at the same time).

The world of vaginoplasty is changing rapidly at the moment, with techniques such as the peritoneal pull-through growing in popularity. Peritoneal techniques utilize material from the lining of the stomach to create the vaginal cavity. As of this writing, these methods are less commonly used than the penile inversion technique, in which the penis and scrotum provide the material for the neovagina. The glans of the penis forms the neoclitoris, so most people who are able to have an orgasm prior to this surgery can have an orgasm after. Penile inversion is less available to women and feminine-spectrum people with smaller penises, who may not be able to obtain the vaginal depth they might want without additional tissue. Penile inversion also does not allow the individual to keep their penis, as the penis is reshaped into the neovagina. With peritoneal techniques the penis can be preserved in its current form if desired, although this is currently a fairly uncommon procedure.

Vaginoplasty currently also necessitates regular dilation of the neovagina in order to retain depth and function. Dilation involves inserting a dilator into the vagina for 15–30 minutes generally three times per day for the first three to six months, twice per day for the next six to nine months, and daily thereafter (although some people have success with weekly dilation starting two years or so after surgery). Dilation is very important to talk about with people considering vaginoplasty, especially those who have experienced sexual trauma. Although I mentioned post-surgical pain as a trigger above, I want to reiterate this here, as dilation is a uniquely invasive—and sometimes uniquely triggering—form of post-surgical care. Talking through the trauma, and planning for the possibility of being triggered by dilation, can go a long way toward managing trauma responses that could increase symptoms of posttraumatic stress disorder, inhibit dilation, or simply increase distress.

SUPPORTING TGD YOUTH

It is truly a tragedy that Republican lawmakers in this country are spending so much of their time and energy persecuting transgender children rather than serving their constituencies. It is also a stain on the nation's character that so many of these constituents welcome the persecution of transgender children as a political position. At the time of this writing, new legislation has either been recently voted into law, or will soon come up for the vote, that restricts the rights of TGD children and youth in 33 states, and in some cases criminalizes medical providers who offer care to TGD children, or opens up the families of TGD children to investigations from the Department of Child and Family Services. This is a shameless, vicious, and coordinated attack on some of the country's least powerful residents. It is also very much in-flux right now—I try to keep up with it on my Medium page (@rminshew) but even that becomes outdated very quickly.

While this book is not about the many conservative "controversies" surrounding TGD children and teens, I want to make sure you have some information available to dispel some of the more common myths surrounding gender diversity in children and adolescents. One of the largest wedge issues seems to be about TGD children competing on gender-segregated sports teams in their affirmed genders. (For a brief overview of why this opportunity is so important for TGD children, see Barrera et al., 2021). While we don't really know all of the ways in which genetics contribute to athletic ability, having XY chromosomes does not seem to confer the amazing athletic advantage that some lawmakers believe it confers. There is evidence to suggest that people with higher testosterone are, at the population level, stronger and faster than people with higher estrogen. (Among elite athletes, however, these data are actually quite mixed.) So, while it may be unfair to teenage girls who are having an estrogen-forward puberty to ask them to compete with someone who is having a testosterone-forward puberty in a sport that centers strength, the way to avoid this is to make space for TGD boys and young men on boys teams not to prohibit TGD girls and young women from participating on girls teams. Moreover, the hypothetical risk that someone with XY chromosomes who is having an uncomplicated testosterone-forward puberty would "fake" being a girl solely in order to be able to compete on a girls' team is an example of a low-probability future theoretical being used to create here-and-now injury to real people.

Another wedge issue is around the gender-affirming treatment model and specifically gonadotropin-hormone releasing agonists and antagonists (sometimes call GnRH blockers or simply "blockers") for children and adolescents. Social transition for young people is similar to that of social transition for adults, in that it might include a different haircut, different clothes, a different name, different pronouns, or all of these. In consultation with the experts at gender clinics, which are medical centers that serve TGD children and youth, some children who want and need it are able to access what is called the "blocker protocol." Gonadotropin releasing hormone analogues prevent the child's body from releasing the endogenous hormones of puberty. They have been used for decades to pause precocious puberty (e.g., puberty beginning before age 8) and are safe and effective for delaying endogenous puberty, by and large with limited other effects (the child's bone density should be monitored, for instance). In gender-related treatment, we talk about blockers as a way of "hitting pause" on puberty so that the child has time to decide if an estrogen-forward or testosterone-forward puberty is right for their body. If a child decides they want the puberty associated with their birth-assigned sex, the blocker can be stopped, and the child will have their endogenous puberty. If the child decides that hormone replacement therapy is right for them, then treatment providers can titrate the blocker and the hormone therapy so that the child goes through different kind of puberty than their body would endogenously allow. Puberty blockers are best offered when a child is at the phase of physical development known as Tanner Stage 2. In Tanner Stage 2, children are just starting puberty, with some minimal growth in genital tissue. This usually begins around age 10 or 11, with the observable changes triggered by the beginning of production of the precursors of endogenous estrogen or testosterone.

When people start blockers at Tanner Stage 2, they don't go through the changes associated with their endogenous puberties. This means that young men and masculine-spectrum people do not develop breasts, and young women and feminine-spectrum people do not do not develop brow ridges or square jaws. For some people, this will mean fewer surgeries as well as, potentially, less persistent or pervasive feelings of gender incongruence. The challenges associated with the blocker protocol and HRT are also associated with pubertal development. Because people who start blockers at Tanner Stage 2 don't have the development associated with their endogenous puberties, their reproductive systems do not develop to the point of producing mature gametes (eggs or sperm). Thus, youth who plan to use the blocker protocol and HRT should receive fertility counseling from a gender-affirming pediatric fertility specialist to talk about how they might want to build families, what level of endogenous pubertal development might be tolerable for them, and the evolving technology of fertility preservation. Another consideration for children born with penises who would like vaginas in the future is that penile inversion vaginoplasty relies on tissue from the penis and scrotum in order to create the neovagina. An adult with a penis and scrotum who used blockers and then had an estrogen-forward puberty might find that they will need additional tissue, although different surgeons differ on their management of this concern.

Puberty is a difficult time of life, whether it's a first or second puberty, and whether it is with hormones that are endogenous or exogenous. Going through a puberty that changes your body in ways that are fundamentally misaligned with your gender identity can be horrifying. The good news is that there is increasing evidence that TGD young people who are supported in their genders are significantly less likely to experience psychological distress than TGD young people who are not supported in their genders (see Ehrensaft et al., 2018, for a review of prepubertal transition).

I almost hate to bring up what is sometimes called rapid onset gender dysphoria (ROGD) because even mentioning it suggests in some way that it is a valid psychological construct. If you have heard about it, or there are parents of young people you treat who are asking you about it, a brief synopsis of the construct is that there is a subset of adolescents (primarily AFAB adolescents) who suddenly decide they are TGD due to peer pressure and the impact of TGD social media influencers.

You should be advised that there are no concrete data to suggest that children are peer-pressured into gender transition. This concept was based on a research paper in which the *parents* of youth who were questioning their gender identities were surveyed (Littman, 2019). The parents surveyed were sampled from sites that are hostile to TGD identities. Guess what? Some parents solicited through online forums with an anti-trans bias had not known their children were questioning their gender identities. Thus, they expressed the belief that their children were succumbing to peer pressure around gender transition when their children did come out. The parents felt their children were moving forward with transition at too-rapid rate, and may be mentally ill rather than TGD. The author of this paper interpreted these data to mean that there is a subset of TGD people who are afflicted with ROGD, were peer-pressured into transition, are vulnerable to peer pressure due to psychopathology, and would come to regret HRT and/or surgery if allowed to access it.

Although post-publication review of this article resulted in a manuscript with an updated title and re-written introduction and conclusion that strongly qualified these conclusions, the construct of ROGD has done a great deal of damage. Indeed, the ROGD argument features heavily in a book about damage—the damage created in impressionable young people if they fall prey to the "transgender craze." Although both the article and book are deeply flawed, they have gained a lot of traction, and I worry that the flawed science and appeals to gender essentialism (or what are sometimes called "gender critical" voices) are compelling at this cultural moment. The preponderance of the evidence disconfirms the existence of ROGD. Most recently, a study of TGD youth examined the relationship between the recency of the youths' understanding of themselves as TGD, and measures of psychopathology and gender dysphoria (Bauer et al., 2021). Youth who more recently understood themselves to be TGD did not endorse more psychopathology, neurodevelopmental disability, maladaptive coping, or indicators of peer influence than youth who had known themselves to be TGD for longer, refuting the hypotheses of the ROGD construct. Unfortunately, this deeply flawed construct has increased parental and provider anxiety about HRT in TGD adolescents.

Certainly, people sometimes experiment with a variety of gender identities and expressions. We should be open to people on any kind of gender journey, including a trajectory in which a person lives for a while in a gender that is different than the gender associated with the person's birth-assigned sex, and then lives for a while (or forever) in the gender associated with their birth-assigned sex. (For a thoughtful and nuanced discussion of this, see Ashley, 2021.) But if we center the understanding that there is no wrong way to do gender, concerns about things like ROGD start to seem rather immaterial.

All of this is perhaps a long-winded way of bringing us back to where we started. Transgender girls are girls. Transgender boys are boys. Nonbinary children are nonbinary. Gender identity and expression might change dramatically over time, or stay more-or-less consistent across the life span. Every person with a body makes decisions about their embodiment goals many times over the course of their lives—and, indeed, throughout an ordinary day. Sometimes these decisions about embodiment goals include deliberation around gender identity and expression. The choices that TGD people make about our bodies are perhaps more deliberative, explicit, and informed than the choices of people whose gender identities and gender expressions are typically associated with their birth-assigned sex. But access to these choices helps create a more vibrant, inclusive, and diverse society for every body, which ultimately benefits everybody.

WORKS CITED

American Psychiatric Association. (1980). *Diagnostic and statistical manual of mental disorders* (3rd edition). American Psychiatric Association.

American Psychiatric Association, & American Psychiatric Association. (2013). *Diagnostic and statistical manual of mental disorders* (5th edition). American Psychiatric Association.

Ashley, F. (2021). The clinical irrelevance of "desistance" research for transgender and gender creative youth. *Psychology of Sexual Orientation and Gender Diversity* (advance electronic publication).

Barrera, E., Millington, K., & Kremen, J. (2021). The medical implications of banning transgender youth from sport participation. *JAMA Pediatrics, 176*(3), 223–224.

Bauer, G. R., Lawson, M. L., Metzger, D. L., & Trans Youth CAN! Research Team. (2021). Do clinical data from transgender adolescents support the phenomenon of "Rapid Onset Gender Dysphoria"?. *The Journal of Pediatrics, 243*, 224–227. E2.

Brownstone, L. M., DeRieux, J., Kelly, D. A., Sumlin, L. J., & Gaudiani, J. L. (2021). Body mass index requirements for gender-affirming surgeries are not empirically based. *Transgender Health, 6*(3), 121–124.

Deutsch, M. B. (Ed.) (2016). *Guidelines for the primary and gender-affirming care of transgender and gender nonbinary people* (2nd edition). UCSF Transgender Care, Department of Family and Community Medicine, University of California San Francisco. Available at transcare.ucsf.edu/guidelines.

Ehrensaft, D. (2017). Gender nonconforming youth: Current perspectives. *Adolescent Health, Medicine and Therapeutics, 8*, 57.

Ehrensaft, D., Giammattei, S. V., Storck, K., Tishelman, A. C., & Keo-Meier, C. (2018). Prepubertal social gender transitions: What we know; what we can learn—A view from a gender affirmative lens. *International Journal of Transgenderism, 19*(2), 251–268.

Ho, F., & Mussap, A. J. (2019). The gender identity scale: Adapting the gender unicorn to measure gender identity. *Psychology of Sexual Orientation and Gender Diversity, 6*(2), 217–231. https://doi.org/10.1037/sgd0000322

James, S. E., Herman, J. L., Rankin, S., Keisling, M., Mottet, L., & Anafi, M. (2016). *The report of the 2015 U.S. transgender survey*. National Center for Transgender Equality.

Keo-Meier, C. E., & Ehrensaft, D. E. (Eds.) (2018). *The gender affirmative model: An interdisciplinary approach to supporting transgender and gender expansive children*. American Psychological Association.

Killermann, S. (2016). The genderbread person. https://www.genderbread.org/resources

Light, A. D., Obedin-Maliver, J., Sevelius, J. M., & Kerns, J. L. (2014). Transgender men who experienced pregnancy after female-to-male gender transitioning. *Obstetrics & Gynecology, 124*(6), 1120–1127.

Littman, L. (2019). Correction: Parent reports of adolescents and young adults perceived to show signs of a rapid onset of gender dysphoria. *PLoS One, 14*(3), e0214157.

McQueen, P. (2017). The role of regret in medical decision-making. *Ethical Theory and Moral Practice, 20*(5), 1051–1065.

Reisner, S. L., Radix, A., & Deutsch, M. B. (2016). Integrated and gender-affirming transgender clinical care and research. *Journal of Acquired Immune Deficiency Syndromes (1999), 72*(Suppl. 3), S235.

Strings, S. (2019). *Fearing the Black body*. New York University Press.

Stryker, S. (2008). *Transgender history*. Seal Press.

Turban, J. L., King, D., Carswell, J. M., & Keuroghlian, A. S. (2020). Pubertal suppression for transgender youth and risk of suicidal ideation. *Pediatrics, 145*(2), e20191725.

van de Grift, T. C., Elaut, E., Cerwenka, S. C., Cohen-Kettenis, P. T., & Kreukels, B. P. (2018). Surgical satisfaction, quality of life, and their association after gender-affirming surgery: A follow-up study. *Journal of Sex & Marital Therapy, 44*(2), 138–148.

World Health Organization. (2018). *International classification of diseases for mortality and morbidity statistics* (11th Revision). WHO.

CHAPTER 2

TRAUMA 101

A BRIEF (AND EUROCENTRIC) DIAGNOSTIC HISTORY OF TRAUMA

The recognition that there is a relationship between trauma exposure and the painful reactivity that emerges in the aftermath of trauma exposure probably goes back to the beginning of the human experience. Life for most people throughout human history has likely had a generous measure of exposure to what we would now call traumatic stress, and presumably families, friends, and community members noticed changes in one another after particularly harrowing experiences. Of course, it is difficult to know precisely, as reactions to stressors only become psychologically "diagnosable" with the creation of a system of psychological diagnosis. But from the very beginning of psychology as a discipline, traumagenic precursors to painful reactivity have been suggested and then disavowed in a predictable cycle.

Sigmund Freud suggested the link between childhood sexual maltreatment and "hysteria" in a theory he called "seduction hypothesis," which he presented in 1896 (see Jones, 1953). But although Freud initially suggested a traumagenic origin of psychological distress, under pressure from the Viennese elite (who apparently did not want to stop abusing their children), he backed off of this position, later asserting that it is the fantasy of childhood sexual maltreatment, rather than the reality of it, that contributes to neurosis. Freud was undoubtedly battling his own demons on this front. He described his father as a sexual abuser in a letter to Wilhelm Fleiss, openly acknowledging his own unwillingness to confront the patriarchs of his era or his own flesh-and-blood patriarch (see Masson, 1985). Instead, he created an interpretation of reality that pleased and placated those patriarchs, as abused children often do. I would call this an enactment that we continue to get stuck in as a society, and this cultural enactment makes it very difficult to talk about the deep and lasting harm of trauma exposure. It is interesting to consider how the field of psychology might look different if it had not been founded by an abused child who had not come to terms with the fallout of his abuse. Or, perhaps, we can speculate: a contemporary of Freud's, Pierre Janet, *did* persist in writing about the negative effects of childhood sexual maltreatment and other forms of childhood maltreatment, maintaining his belief that maltreatment and mental illness are inextricably tied (see Brown & Van der Horst, 1998). He also wrote about the relationship between abuse and dissociative symptoms (see Van der Hart & Horst, 1989). It is telling that his work was sidelined in favor of theories that fit the status quo rather than the data. I would argue that our systems of medicine, including psychological medicine, are either ultimately co-opted by the interests of the powerful, or are invisibilized and defamed as not credible when they aren't co-opted.

The relationship between traumatic experiences on the battlefield and quantifiable psychological sequelae was formally noted during the First World War, as more and more soldiers started returning home with what was then called shell shock. Charles Myers reported on this phenomenon in *The Lancet* (1915). It is interesting to observe some of the differences in presentation of shell shock and what we now think of as trauma-related sequelae—most notably that the disruptions of shell shock were located in the body, in the form of muscular weakness and nerve pain, rather than in the mind. This suggests that, although responses to

DOI: 10.4324/9781003140740-3

traumatic stressors happen across times and cultures, the ways in which trauma responses *present* are at least partly socially constructed. It also provides an important springboard for a range of contemporary theories of traumatic stress, which suggest that trauma is held in the body as least as much as in the mind. We'll be revisiting some of these theories in Chapters 5 and 10.

Posttraumatic stress disorder (PTSD) was formalized in contemporary diagnostic nosology in 1980, in the same version of the *Diagnostic and Statistical Manual of Mental Disorders* (DSM) that introduced "transsexualism" (third edition, 1980). (I'll mention here that the word transsexual is a dated term that should not be used in contemporary clinical practice.) The PTSD diagnosis was developed to describe the experience of American veterans of the American War in Vietnam. Because it was created to describe the experience of soldiers returning from combat, it centered a particular experience of trauma. The exposure criteria regarding what qualified as a traumatic stressor were limited to what were considered extraordinary events such as exposure to combat or natural disaster.

Trauma-related diagnostic categories have continued to evolve, and there are debates in the field about what trauma-related diagnoses should and shouldn't incorporate as well as a growing recognition of the range of individual differences in reaction to trauma exposure. The first questions of this kind were articulated by Judith Herman in her groundbreaking *Trauma and Recovery: The Aftermath of Violence—From Domestic Abuse to Political Terror* (1992). Although couched in the language of a binary formulation of gender (in a time in which the word nonbinary was not used to describe gender identity) her focus on "women's trauma" centered traumatic sequelae in the aftermath of violence that takes place in homes and communities, including homes and communities that are far from battlefields and war rooms. Herman was also clear that, for large swaths of the population, including cisgender women and children, home is by far the most dangerous environment. At the center of her book was a simple premise: different people have different experiences with trauma exposure, and these differences in experiences (1) are sometimes predicated on identity factors and (2) might result in different symptom profiles. This premise establishes a range of questions about the diagnosis of posttraumatic sequelae that have not been fully answered at the time of this writing. A person who is chronically abused at home, for instance, may never experience fear of death in that context or sustain life-threatening injury. This person may also not experience flashbacks or what a diagnostician would consider intrusive memories. Thus, this person would not meet either the exposure or symptom criteria of PTSD. If, instead, this person is chronically dissociative and experiences themself as unlovable, does this person have a trauma-related disorder? If not, how do we understand their symptom profile? If so, how do we distinguish between this type of trauma-related disorder and PTSD? Should we expand what it means to have PTSD? Establish a different trauma-related diagnosis? Or reify the symptoms of PTSD as a threshold to which trauma-related reactions must rise in order to be a diagnosable trauma-related condition?

Those who suggest that there should be different diagnoses that capture sequelae relative to different types of trauma exposure argue that the narrow inclusion and symptom criteria of PTSD, while describing a particular manifestation of posttraumatic sequelae, implicitly disavow the experiences of people who are injured by experiences such as some forms of childhood maltreatment, psychological abuse, and some forms of chronic trauma. If there are no trauma-related diagnoses that capture this experience, this position maintains, individuals with these trauma-related symptoms remain undiagnosed, or garner a range of seemingly unrelated diagnoses in an effort to categorize and treat symptoms related to their experiences, without ever explicitly identifying the experiences as the trigger for the problem (see, e.g., van der Kolk et al., 2009). Scientists and clinicians on this side of the debate have, over the years, proposed other trauma disorders that might be added to the DSM in order to better describe the sequelae of ongoing traumatic stress that may never cause a person to fear for their life. This push started with a proposal for a condition called Disorders of Extreme Stress Not Otherwise Specified (DESNOS), and ultimately progressed to a proposal for a condition called Developmental Trauma Disorder (DTD), both of which center dissociation as a prominent trauma-related symptom. While none of the developmental trauma diagnoses have been codified in the DSM as of this writing, the fifth edition has instead broadened the exposure criterion for PTSD, and also added a specifier for a Dissociative Subtype of PTSD, in order to better incorporate this range of profiles. The *International Statistical Classification of Diseases and Related Health Problems* (ICD-11; World Health Organization, 2019), on the other hand, has gone a different route, opting to identify two sibling diagnoses, PTSD and complex posttraumatic stress disorder (CPTSD) in an effort to add nuance and diagnostic flexibility for trauma-based symptoms. Although there continues to be debate regarding the utility of the CPTSD diagnosis, a recent review of the literature pertaining to a specific trauma questionnaire (the International Trauma Questionnaire) found consistent support for discriminability between the symptoms of PTSD and CPTSD (Redican et al., 2021). Moreover, as the diagnostic category of CPTSD was in the process of consideration for ICD-11, a number of studies that focused on discriminant validity (e.g., Ben-Ezra et al., 2018), the factor structure (e.g., Hansen et al., 2015), the second-order factor structure (e.g., Hyland et al., 2017), and population-level base rates of PTSD versus CPTSD were conducted, further establishing a base of empirical support for the sibling diagnoses.

On the other side of the debate, those who advocate for a single diagnosis of PTSD (with the inclusion of modifiers as necessary to capture an individual's unique symptom profile) suggest that the evidence to support a CPTSD diagnostic category is insufficient (e.g., Resick et al., 2012). Moreover, those who hold this position argue, there is already a diagnostic category that captures the symptom profile of CPTSD: that of borderline personality disorder (BPD). Someone might have both PTSD and BPD, and in that case should be diagnosed with both PTSD and BPD rather than creating a new diagnostic category. This is the more clinically relevant formulation, this position asserts, as treatments for both PTSD and BPD (and co-occurring PTSD and BPD) already exist. Diagnosing someone in a new diagnostic category, for which there is not the same body of literature of empirically validated treatment studies, may lead to more suffering on the part of people with these diagnoses. For instance, a person may reject treatments for PTSD and BPD because they have a diagnosis of CPTSD, and then feel their symptom constellation is "too complex" to treat in a meaningful way because there are fewer treatment guidelines for CPTSD. Finally, this position suggests, discriminating between PTSD and CPTSD may extend the suffering of people diagnosed with CPTSD, as treatment for CPTSD typically incorporates a phase of safety and stabilization. The safety and stabilization phase not only prolongs treatment overall, but it also delays the onset of the exposure portion of treatment, which has the strongest evidence base, potentially harming the individual or prolonging their suffering (e.g., De Jongh et al., 2016).

As this manuscript favors a phase-based approach to treatment, my biases on this particular question are probably clear: I think the CPTSD diagnosis has utility and should be incorporated into our system of diagnosis insofar as we utilize a diagnostic system, and I'm onboard with the ever-growing body of literature that indicates that the sibling diagnoses are discriminable from one another and also may require different treatment strategies (see, e.g., Cloitre, 2021). While I acknowledge my particular bias, I also acknowledge that the questions surrounding phase-based treatments are legitimate, and different clinicians of good will and intention may come down on different sides of the debate regarding the utility of a safety and stabilization phase of treatment. If you feel that phase-based treatment is unnecessary or unethical, I hope that Chapter 11, which is focused on reprocessing and has a lengthy discussion of exposure-based methods, will have some use for you.

At first glance, the question of the number of trauma-related diagnoses may seem purely academic, or a question that perhaps impacts diagnosis, but not really treatment. But there are many reasons why this diagnostic question has been so hotly contested. For one, understanding causality can, in fact, be very important for appropriate treatment of symptoms. A classic paper underscoring the importance of this distinction was a study of chronic depression, with an eye toward assessing the treatment efficacy of antidepressants alone, psychotherapy alone, and a combination of antidepressants and psychotherapy (Nemeroff et al., 2003). The data indicated that the combination of antidepressant medication and psychotherapy was more effective than antidepressants alone or psychotherapy alone, and that the monotherapies of either psychotherapy or an antidepressant were approximately equal in their effects. However, when the participants were stratified by childhood trauma exposure, a different pattern of results emerged. The people in the study who had experienced early childhood trauma benefitted significantly more from psychotherapy alone than antidepressant therapy alone, and there was only a small effect of combining psychotherapy with an antidepressant. In other words, the therapy was the crucial element for the group with exposure to childhood trauma, while the antidepressant carried the effect for the group without exposure to childhood trauma. There are a couple of important things to bear in mind about this study. First, this was a study of depression, not PTSD, CPTSD, or developmental trauma, so the participants in this study were involved in the study because they met the criteria of major depressive disorder (MDD). Second, the group was stratified based on childhood trauma exposure, not on specifically trauma-related symptoms such as intrusive thoughts or hyperarousal. In other words, the researchers would not necessarily have had reason to believe that their participants had exposure to childhood trauma *per se*, even though about 60% of the participants did in fact have this exposure. To my mind, this suggests that when someone comes to our offices with MDD (or generalized anxiety disorder, or bipolar disorder, and especially when people carry multiple diagnoses), we should start with the hypothesis that trauma exposure may be involved in etiology, even if it takes some time for us to confirm or disconfirm this hypothesis.

Another reason why granular diagnosis of trauma-related symptomatology can be important is that, in psychology, granular diagnosis also guides research opportunities. It is very difficult to obtain grants for a condition that is not in the DSM or ICD, and grants are currently the mechanism by which we are able to develop a research-based understanding of a disorder. To the best of my knowledge, this has changed somewhat with the Research Domain Criteria Initiative (RDoC), launched in 2009 by the National Institute of Mental Health. RDoC focuses on domains of functioning, rather than diagnoses, for adjudicating grant funding. (For an overview of some of the contributions and gaps related to RDoC-centered research on PTSD, see Schmidt & Vermetten (2018). It could be that continued focus on domains of functioning, rather than diagnostic categories, will ultimately recenter the research literature.

Our granular system of diagnosis also undergirds insurance compensation for psychological treatment. A DSM or ICD diagnosis is required as part of insurance billing paperwork, and sometimes the type of treatment that can be offered to someone seeking services is contingent on the diagnosis. This has the potential to be harmful when someone needs trauma-informed treatment due to, say, early childhood trauma, but does not meet criteria for PTSD and is instead presenting with symptoms more consistent with generalized anxiety disorder. Ethical clinicians might find themselves caught between the desire to accurately diagnose and efficaciously treat, or having to disqualify an individual from services at a specialty trauma clinic because their trauma does not meet Criterion A.

With all of this said, I'll also acknowledge that I am also no longer fully convinced that the PTSD-versus-sibling-diagnoses-of-PTSD-and-CPTSD debate is the central diagnostic question regarding traumatic sequelae. My thoughts and perspectives on this have shifted as I have had the opportunity to think more conceptually about our system of diagnosis and specifically about diagnoses related to gender diversity and neurodiversity. If we center diversity, equity, and inclusion, instead of seeing them as peripheral, it becomes evident that there are some big problems in categorizing some experiences as "bad enough" to warrant support, while others are implicitly deemed "not that bad" and thus support is withheld. There is also an element of paternalism in deciding that this or that reaction to a traumatic or stressful experience is a symptom, while another reaction is "normal" or "healthy." People are having the experiences they are having, and these are partially manifestations of the experiences that they have had before. If the experiences they are having right now are causing them anguish or discomfort, they should have access to needed supports—not so they can become "normal" or have a "subthreshold clinical presentation" but so they can be supported. There is not really much space in this perspective for the use of a diagnostic system, no matter how refined, to adjudicate who "qualifies" for needed supports. However, since we do currently operate within a diagnostic system, an understanding of diagnostic nosology is important, and thus described below. (One hope that I have is that an understanding of psychiatric diagnostic nosology can become a framework for the subversion of psychiatric diagnostic nosology, but that is an area for future research.)

THE DIAGNOSTIC CRITERIA

According to the DSM-V, PTSD can be diagnosed if the individual had exposure to "actual or threatened death, serious injury, or sexual violence" themselves or (in some cases) secondarily. This is the exposure criterion or Criterion A. Following this exposure, an individual must report at least one symptom of intrusion related to the event, which might include persistent memories or dreams, flashbacks, or marked reactivity to cues associated with the traumatic stressor (Criterion B). They must also experience marked effort to avoid internal or external reminders of the stressor (Criterion C). Additionally, they must report at least two "negative alterations in mood or cognition," which might include diminished interest in activities, negative beliefs about self or others, dissociative amnesia, or inability to experience positive emotions (Criterion D). If these symptoms persist for more than a month, and significantly impact a person's functioning, a diagnosis of PTSD is warranted.

In ICD-11, the sibling diagnoses of PTSD and CPTSD share a similar etiology, in that they arise as reactions to "extremely threatening or horrific" events. PTSD can be diagnosed, according to ICD-11 classification, if the individual reports intrusive memories of the event, avoidance of reminders of the event, and increased threat reactivity such as hypervigilance or increased startle reflex in the wake of the event. CPTSD can be diagnosed when the exposure to "extremely threatening or horrific events" is ongoing, repetitive, and there is no possibility of escape. CPTSD is characterized by the three core symptoms of PTSD and three additional symptom clusters called Disturbances of

Self-Organization (DSOs). The symptoms clusters specific to the DSOs are affective dys-regulation, negative self-concept, and relationship difficulties. While CPTSD was being studied as a construct, DSOs were assessed with questions from standardized measures that had face validity for measuring these constructs. More recently, the International Trauma Questionnaire (ITQ) has been tested and validated as a measure for assessing PTSD and CPTSD, and disambiguating between the two (Cloitre et al., 2018).

The re-experiencing criterion of both PTSD and CPTSD is assessed on the ITQ with eight questions related to intrusive memories of the stressor, including memories that lead the person to feel as if the stressor is happening in the here-and-now. These questions include assessment of disturbing dreams about the stressor, flashbacks, or moments of extreme reaction to a reminder of the stressor followed by spacing out or shutting down. The avoidance criterion of both PTSD and CPTSD is assessed on the ITQ with two questions regarding the avoidance of trauma reminders. One question focuses on internal avoidance (e.g., avoiding thoughts or sensations related to the stressor) and one question on external avoidance (e.g., avoiding similar locations to which the stressor took place). The threat-reactivity criterion of both PTSD and CPTSD is assessed on the ITQ with two questions, one that assesses guardedness and one that assesses "jumpiness" or startle reflex. These criteria form the core diagnostic criteria of both PTSD and CPTSD.

The affective dysregulation criterion of CPTSD is assessed in the ITQ using nine questions related to emotional responding. Five of these questions speak to the experience of hyperreactivity: these include feeling easily hurt and experiences of uncontrollable anger. The remaining four questions speak to hyporeactivity, such as numbing, or the feeling of being outside one's body. A study that sought to further understand the affective dysregulation symptom cluster used confirmatory factor analysis to indicate that affective dysregulation can be best conceptualized as bidimensional, with domains of hypoactivation and hyperactivation (Karatzias et al., 2018). It should be noted, then, that an individual with CPTSD might be high in both of these dimensions, reporting both more emotional hyper-activation and also more emotional hypoactivation than control groups. Those of us who work clinically with individuals who either meet CPTSD criteria or who have experienced significant trauma and stress observe that it is common for individuals with these experiences to toggle rapidly between hyper-and hypoactivity, spending little or no time in a state of "just right" activation to meet the current moment. These observations have resulted in theories related to the so-called window of tolerance, which will be revisited in Chapters 5 and 10.

The second DSO cluster is negative self-concept. Negative self-concept is assessed on the ITQ with four questions related to feelings about the self, including feelings of shame and worthlessness. A recent study indicates that self-compassion is low in people with CPTSD, and particularly in those high in negative self-concept (Karatzias et al., 2019). In this study, the construct of self-compassion explained almost 30% of the variance in symptoms related to negative self-concept. This suggests yet another avenue for treating CPTSD, namely, using therapeutic strategies to build self-compassion.

The final DSO cluster is difficulty with relationships. This is assessed on the ITQ with three questions related to relationships, including feeling cut off from others, and difficulty staying close with others. Some people who struggle in this domain find that they are isolated and alone, protecting themselves from pain and disappointment by protecting themselves from the messy intimacy of human relationships. Others find themselves in relationships that burn fast and hot, rapidly forming friendships (often built around sharing about a lot of information about traumatic experiences very quickly) that flare up and flame out before they can ever really become safe and comfortable. From my perspective, the relationships

DSO presents the clearest clinical evidence for why a slower, phase-based trauma treatment is crucial when working with CPTSD. A relationship with a therapist is a significant relationship. When there is time pressure to share about trauma with a clinician, we can wind up in a replication process with our vulnerable clients that simply does not serve them, becoming another one of those hot-and-fast relationships that explodes or disappears. This also indicates that therapists must become comfortable slowing down disclosures when clients may want to rush into them in harmful ways. Strategies for evaluating this, and slowing down when necessary, are discussed in Chapter 11.

These are currently the ways in which traumas are diagnosed and categorized: through the DSM-V criteria of PTSD, or the ICD-11 criteria of PTSD and CPTSD. So, in order to place someone in a trauma-based diagnostic category, we continue to look for the key components of "significant" trauma, intrusive memories, avoidance, and hypervigilance. We then expand from here either with specifiers or through assessing for DSOs. But what constitutes a "significant" trauma? And whose evaluation of what is "significant" should we center?

In this manuscript, I center the experiences, notably the traumatic and stressful experiences, of TGD people. And while TGD people are assaulted, sexually assaulted, and murdered at higher rates than the general population, being shamed, humiliated, unwitnessed, and unloved by the people who are supposed to care about us can sometimes be more injurious to us than other forms of aggression. Moreover, these are the kinds of experiences that encourage people to try to hide and disguise who they are, to feel ashamed of who they are, and to feel like maybe they deserve the bad things that happen to them. When we feel like we deserve bad things, there's certainly no shortage of bad things out there to find us, and the trauma begins to "load." And when other people believe we deserve bad things, these experiences cannot be held in community, and recovery becomes exponentially more difficult. So, while I do think it's important to be conversant with the diagnostic criteria of our field, I would argue that other kinds of stressors, and other kinds of sequelae, are equally important in the lives of TGD people. Thus, the rest of this chapter will be devoted to outlining different theories and definitions of trauma, stress, and stigma. Adverse childhood experiences (ACEs), microaggressions, institutional trauma, and moral injury, are discussed below. We'll then discuss some of the unifying theories of minority stress and stigma that draw links between the biological and the social in terms of understanding trauma- and stress-related psychological difficulties.

ADVERSE CHILDHOOD EXPERIENCES

A discussion of trauma and stress would be incomplete without a section devoted to Felitti and colleagues' seminal study of ACEs (Felitti et al., 1998). Originally designed as a health behaviors and health outcomes study, the ACEs study explicated the link between difficult experiences in childhood, and health behaviors and health outcomes in adults. The original ACEs study consisted of a ten-question questionnaire including questions about abuse (physical, emotional, and sexual), neglect (physical and emotional), and metrics of household dysfunction such as living with someone with mental illness or drug addiction, witnessing domestic violence, having an incarcerated relative, or experiencing the divorce of parents. This questionnaire was dispatched to 13,494 individuals who had recently completed a health evaluation and were insured through a large HMO (Kaiser Permanente). More than 9,000 individuals responded to the questionnaire and also allowed researchers access to their health behaviors and outcomes information as assessed through the HMO. The outcomes of the ACEs study were clear: there was a graded relationship between number of adverse experiences in childhood and adult diseases, including cardiac incidents, hypertension, chronic pain, kidney disease, mental illness, diabetes, and sexually transmitted infection. People with four or more ACEs were more than 12 times more likely to have attempted suicide than those with no ACEs and four times more likely to have experienced depression in the last year.

The original ACEs study included a preponderance of individuals who were white and middle-class, and of course every individual in the original study had health insurance (as they were recruited via their insurer). There were also no questions about gender identity or expression—female and male were the demographic options for reporting sex assigned at birth, and gender was not asked about as a separate entity from sex assigned at birth. The results of the study were robust and significant enough, however, to trigger a proliferation of studies on ACEs and health outcomes, and the development of an internationally recognized tool for measuring ACEs that captures global experiences of childhood (the WHO's Adverse Childhood Experiences International Questionnaire, 2018. See also Struck et al., 2021, for an overview of ACEs-inspired manuscripts). Moreover, the lens of ACEs has been expanded to incorporate common experiences of American children that were not captured by the preliminary ACE study by expanding the definition of ACEs and sampling broader populations (e.g., Cronholm et al., 2015). Some studies include community-level stressors (e.g., Wade et al., 2016) and global stressors (such as climate change) as ACEs, and together, these have informed the dialogue around what is called toxic stress. It should be noted, however, that the vast majority of these studies retain the male-female binary when asking for demographic information (see Schnarrs et al., 2019, for an exception to this rule—this study will also be discussed in more detail in Chapter 4).

Felitti and colleagues' primary understanding of the link between ACEs and health concerns was health behaviors. Children experiencing ACEs might turn to coping strategies such as smoking, food, alcohol, and sex, to manage feelings related to ACEs, thereby increasing the risk of heart disease, diabetes, liver disease, and sexually transmitted infection. A critique of the ACEs literature expands this model to incorporate research on the biology of early adversity as well as the social determinants of health (McEwen & Gregerson, 2019). Models of minority stress, described below, can offer unifying biopsychosocial theories for understanding these differences.

Are ACEs Criterion A stressors? That depends. Some forms of physical and sexual maltreatment would certainly be considered Criterion A stressors, while in most cases, emotional maltreatment and various forms of neglect would not. Living with a person who has been incarcerated would not necessarily be considered a Criterion A stressor; however, an experience of a police raid in which someone is violently removed from the home and other members of the household fear for their lives could be a Criterion A stressor.

MICROAGGRESSIONS

The word microaggression was introduced to contemporary psychology in the work of Sue and colleagues (they credit Pierce, 1970, with the term and original description), who described racial microaggressions as brief interactions that communicate racial slights or insults (Sue et al., 2007). These everyday acts of violence, typically aimed at BIPOC by white people, are often keenly felt by those who are aggressed-against, while generally just on the "deniable" side of the line of plausible deniability for the aggressors. Indeed, the aggressor may not have been cognizant of communicating biases, or even that they have these biases, and thus will sometimes gaslight the aggressed-against by calling them "too sensitive." Sue and colleagues described three different types of racial microaggressions: microassaults, microinsults, and microinvalidations. Microassaults tend to be the most visible, typically reflect consciously held beliefs that are purposively communicated. These may take the form of name-calling or easily recognizable avoidance (e.g., a white server serving a BIPOC customer last despite the customers' order of arrival). Microinsults are more subtle communications such as visibly disengaging when a BIPOC individual is speaking and thereby suggesting their contributions are less valuable. Microinvalidations occur when others question the reality or validity of an individual's experience of racism or in some way question an individual's belongingness through race-based stereotypes.

While Sue and colleagues' work initially focused on racial microaggressions, this framework has been extended to explore microaggressions experienced by sexual and gender minorities (e.g., Nadal, 2018), disabled people (e.g., Kattari, 2020), poor people (e.g., Locke & Trolian, 2018), and religious minorities (e.g., Cheng et al., 2019). Studies have examined microaggressions in academic contexts, the workplace, and the therapy office, among others. There is also a TGD-specific literature on experiences of microaggressions, which will be discussed in more detail in Chapter 4. Microaggressions have been associated with depression, anxiety, and negative affect (e.g., Nadal et al., 2014). Microaggressions have also been linked to disparities in physical health (e.g., Nadal et al., 2017). Microaggressions would not typically qualify as a Criterion A stressor and thus would not result in a PTSD or CPTSD diagnosis no matter how frequent or egregious. By some measurements of ACEs, some microaggressions could be assessed as ACEs.

INSTITUTIONAL BETRAYAL

In the editorial opening of an edition of the *Journal of Trauma and Dissociation*, editors Smidt and Freyd describe institutional betrayal as taking place on two axes and thus across four quadrants (2018). One of the axes they identify is the axis of type of institutional betrayal, with acts of commission and acts of omission. The other axis they describe as the pertaining to the original apparent problem, and whether it is seemingly systemic or seemingly isolated. Although institutions can fail anyone who relies on them for support (which is all of us, at many different points in our lives), there are some specific ways in which institutions betray TGD people. While I'm sure there are other examples, I'll briefly mention some of the institutions that fail to protect TGD people (through acts of commission and acts of omission). While detention facilities such as jails, prisons, and immigration detention fail everyone, they have some particular failures when it comes to TGD people. TGD people are also injured by religious institutions, educational institutions, the military, and the medical system (including the systems of psychology and psychiatry). This list will be revisited in more detail in Chapter 4.

MORAL INJURY

There is a growing body of literature regarding what is called moral injury, which is sometimes defined as perpetrating, or in some way participating in, acts that violate strongly held moral beliefs. A recent review of the moral injury literature, which has focused primarily on military combatants, suggests that moral injury contributes to symptoms of PTSD, depression, and non-suicidal self-injury (Griffin et al., 2019). Additional areas of research into moral injury include moral injury among adolescents (see Kidwell & Keurig, 2021) and moral injury in people who work for Child Protective Services and also in system-involved parents (see Haight et al., 2017).

I'm not sure if the moral injury framework is the best one for the phenomenon I'm reflecting on in this section, but it does capture at least a part of what I observe in my clinical practice. While it is extremely difficult and painful to have been victimized, some of the most difficult clinical work is around acceptance of the places in which we have been *victimizers*. While we acknowledge that the intergenerational transmission of trauma is an empirically grounded phenomenon and can conceptually grasp that hurt people hurt people, many of us are unprepared for what this means in working with trauma survivors. What it means is that we are also working with perpetrators. Moreover, it means that we have to find a way to tolerate our clients' acts of perpetration; otherwise, they will not be able to talk with us about those acts nor will they be able to come to terms with those acts in themselves. And when those acts remain splintered off and intolerable, this, in my experience, heightens the risk for additional perpetration.

As far as I'm aware there is not solid research data about perpetration by TGD people, or moral injury in TGD people who are not also veterans. But because I am aware that this type of perpetration does happen, and because coming to terms with being a perpetrator can be one of the hardest parts of trauma work, I want to speak to this lacuna in the literature, and will discuss this further in Chapter 4.

MODELS OF UNDERSTANDING TRAUMA AND RELATED SYMPTOMATOLOGY

The minority stress model was initially posited as a mechanism for understanding health disparities in sexual minority populations, particularly lesbians (Brooks, 1981; I did not know this until I read Rich et al., 2020). The original model includes multiple levels of stressors, while the more contemporary overview suggests that there are three mechanisms by which minority stress contributes to mental health disparities in LGB populations (Meyer, 2003). First is through direct lived experience of anti-LGB bias such as discrimination or violence. Second is through the experience of vigilance (or hypervigilance) due to the expectation of rejection or discrimination based on anti-LGB bias. The third is through the internalization of anti-LGB biases and attitudes, resulting in internalized homophobia. The minority stress model is frequently used as an organizing framework for understanding health disparities in sexual and gender minority populations. While the original model was constructed around sexual minorities, it was extended to TGD populations, with a bit of variation (e.g., the internalization of anti-trans bias as separate from bias related to sexual identity; Hendricks & Testa, 2012). A recent review of studies related to TGD mental health disparities assess more than 70 research articles with TGD populations in order to identify gaps in the literature, and used the MSM as a unifying framework for identifying these gaps (Valentine & Shipherd, 2018). Another model focuses more on structural stigma rather than internal processes and makes the important point that community-level stigma is a moderator of therapeutic efficacy (Hatzenbuehler, 2016). Although the Meyer model of minority stress is perhaps more widely used in public health research than the structural model of stigma,

I tend to center structural stigma in my own formulations of TGD trauma and stress. For a review of stigma-related studies specifically focused on TGD people (rather than sexual minorities) see King et al. (2020).

TRAUMA DIAGNOSIS VERSUS TRAUMA-CENTERED FRAME

All of the aforementioned stratifications, from Criterion A stressors through to the trauma of perpetration, are simply theoretical classifications of different kinds of experiences that people have. It can be helpful to view these types of experiences through the lens of classification because recognizing trauma, stress, and systemic oppression can also help us be aware of some of the more typical human reactions to trauma, stress, and systemic oppression. When we are able to recognize the wide ranges of reactions to trauma, we can also begin to identify unifying themes. As we'll discuss in future chapters, we can also develop hypotheses about the biological and psychological concomitants of what we might call psychopathology. Moreover, we can begin to test hypotheses about the kind of interventions that might be helpful for shifting trauma reactions, if a person decides they want those reactions to shift. (Not everyone does want their reactions to shift, and that is also a valid life choice. But as some of these reactions can be quite uncomfortable, many people *do* want them to shift, and benefit from guidance when working to shift them.)

Is an experience that empirically *was* life-threatening more of a Criterion A stressor than something that *felt* life-threatening? What if the person whose life was threatened never develops symptoms of PTSD, and the other person does? How do we define trauma exposure, and is it important to do so? Does it matter if we think about one particular type of difficult experience as "trauma" and another as "stress"? Clinicians vary on this metric. The way I navigate this larger question is by centering the reactions rather than the definitions, and being guided by my clients regarding which reactions they want to work through. Understanding diagnostic nosology has helped me recognize that trauma-based reactions have some common patterns. This makes it easier for me to recognize those reactions as they are manifesting in my clients, which then helps me to share this information with my clients. Sometimes, simply sharing this information can help someone feel less scared by their reactions, and even start to see the ways in which those reactions were helpful to them at difficult times in their lives. Numbing out in day-to-day life, for instance, can feel very alarming. When we recognize it as a trauma reaction and acknowledge how useful it has been for coping with trauma, it can start to feel less like a big, scary, unspeakable problem, and more like an effective coping strategy for a past experience, although one that is unhelpful at the moment.

A question that arises from time-to-time is whether I put too much emphasis on traumatic and stressful experiences. It's possible that I do. If I do, it may be coming from a place of overcorrection, as I have found it to be exceedingly rare for people to initially place much weight in difficult lived experiences as drivers of mental health concerns. Clients will tell me that an experience "wasn't that bad" or explain to me that they "shouldn't" feel as upset about something as they do. Clinicians will tell me that they don't really ask about trauma history. People on airplanes will knock back their third cocktail before telling me that they endured harsh physical discipline as children and "turned out just fine." Indeed, the majority of people I have encountered in clinical settings (yes, airplanes count) do not give trauma much conscious space at all. Trauma is difficult and painful to think about. Just ask Freud.

Moreover, when I *have* seen patients and clients center trauma in their understanding of their own reactivity, I have sometimes also seen mental health providers dismiss or ignore this centering. One of the first patients I ever encountered was at rounds during my first year of clinical training, in which I completed practicum on the inpatient unit of a hospital. The patient, a middle-aged Black cisgender man diagnosed with schizophrenia, finished almost every sentence by telling us that he had been sexually assaulted. The attending physician did not comment on this disclosure in any way and instead simply continued to ask the patient questions intended to establish his orientation to time and place. The patient compliantly responded with answers about the date, the name of the president, etc., but at the end of every answer, he would reiterate, "you know, I was raped. I think maybe I feel so bad because I was raped." At the end of this intake, he was prescribed a higher dose of antipsychotic medication and escorted back to the day room, without having the nexus of his pain attended to or even witnessed. All of which is to say that whether we call an experience trauma or stress or bias or oppression is all one to me. What I believe is important is recognizing the sequelae that accompany it, and being able to ask about and abide with these experiences in order to reduce the harm they are causing. If pressed, my definition of trauma would be that it is anything that overwhelms the organism's capacity to cope to such an extent that the experience contributes to non-flexible reactivity that is not adaptive to the current environment. When we are able to bring down physiological reactivity and understand psychological reactivity, we are able to select from a much broader array of behavioral choices, which I would center as the goal of trauma treatment.

WORKS CITED

American Psychiatric Association. (1980). *Diagnostic and statistical manual of mental disorders* (3rd edition). American Psychiatric Association.

American Psychiatric Association. (2013). *Diagnostic and statistical manual of mental disorders* (5th edition). American Psychiatric Association.

Ben-Ezra, M., Karatzias, T., Hyland, P., Brewin, C. R., Cloitre, M., Bisson, J. I., … Shevlin, M. (2018). Posttraumatic stress disorder (PTSD) and complex PTSD (CPTSD) as per ICD-11 proposals: A population study in Israel. *Depression and Anxiety, 35*(3), 264–274.

Brooks, V. R. (1981). *Minority stress and lesbian women*. Free Press.

Brown, P., & Van der Hart, O. (1998). Memories of sexual abuse: Janet's critique of Freud, a balanced approach. *Psychological Reports, 82*(3), 1027–1043.

Cheng, Z. H., Pagano Jr, L. A., & Shariff, A. F. (2019). The development, validation, and clinical implications of the Microaggressions Against Religious Individuals Scale (MARIS). *Psychology of Religion and Spirituality, 11*(4), 327.

Cloitre, M. (2021). Complex PTSD: Assessment and treatment. *European Journal of Psychotraumatology, 12*(Suppl. 1), 1866423.

Cloitre, M., Shevlin, M., Brewin, C. R., Bisson, J. I., Roberts, N. P., Maercker, A., … Hyland, P. (2018). The International Trauma Questionnaire: Development of a self-report measure of ICD-11 PTSD and complex PTSD. *Acta Psychiatrica Scandinavica, 138*(6), 536–546.

Cronholm, P. F., Forke, C. M., Wade, R., Bair-Merritt, M. H., Davis, M., Harkins-Schwarz, M., … Fein, J. A. (2015). Adverse childhood experiences: Expanding the concept of adversity. *American Journal of Preventive Medicine, 49*(3), 354–361.

De Jongh, A. D., Resick, P. A., Zoellner, L. A., Van Minnen, A., Lee, C. W., Monson, C. M., … Bicanic, I. A. (2016). Critical analysis of the current treatment guidelines for complex PTSD in adults. *Depression and Anxiety, 33*(5), 359–369.

Felitti, V. J., Anda, R. F., Nordenberg, D., Williamson, D. F., Spitz, A. M., Edwards, V., & Marks, J. S. (1998). Relationship of childhood abuse and household dysfunction to many of the leading causes of death in adults: The Adverse Childhood Experiences (ACE) Study. *American Journal of Preventive Medicine, 14*(4), 245–258.

Griffin, B. J., Purcell, N., Burkman, K., Litz, B. T., Bryan, C. J., Schmitz, M., … Maguen, S. (2019). Moral injury: An integrative review. *Journal of Traumatic Stress, 32*(3), 350–362.

Haight, W., Sugrue, E., Calhoun, M., & Black, J. (2017). Everyday coping with moral injury: The perspectives of professionals and parents involved with child protection services. *Children and Youth Services Review, 82*, 108–121.

Hansen, M., Hyland, P., Armour, C., Shevlin, M., & Elklit, A. (2015). Less is more? Assessing the validity of the ICD-11 model of PTSD across multiple trauma samples. *European Journal of Psychotraumatology, 6*, 28766.

Hatzenbuehler, M. L. (2016). Structural stigma: Research evidence and implications for psychological science. *American Psychologist, 71*(8), 742.

Hendricks, M. L., & Testa, R. J. (2012). A conceptual framework for clinical work with transgender and gender nonconforming clients: An adaptation of the Minority Stress Model. *Professional Psychology: Research and Practice, 43*(5), 460.

Herman, J. L. (1992). *Trauma and recovery: The aftermath of violence from domestic abuse to political terror.* BasicBooks.

Hyland, P., Shevlin, M., Brewin, C. R., Cloitre, M., Downes, A. J., Jumbe, S., … Roberts, N. P. (2017). Validation of post-traumatic stress disorder (PTSD) and complex PTSD using the International Trauma Questionnaire. *Acta Psychiatrica Scandinavica, 136*(3), 313–322.

Jones, E. (1953). *The life and work of Sigmund Freud.* Basic Books.

Karatzias, T., Hyland, P., Ben-Ezra, M., & Shevlin, M. (2018). Hyperactivation and hypoactivation affective dysregulation symptoms are integral in complex posttraumatic stress disorder: Results from a nonclinical Israeli sample. *International Journal of Methods in Psychiatric Research, 27*(4), e1745.

Karatzias, T., Hyland, P., Bradley, A., Fyvie, C., Logan, K., Easton, P., … Shevlin, M. (2019). Is self-compassion a worthwhile therapeutic target for ICD-11 complex PTSD (CPTSD)? *Behavioural and Cognitive Psychotherapy, 47*(3), 257–269.

Kattari, S. K. (2020). Ableist microaggressions and the mental health of disabled adults. *Community Mental Health Journal, 56*(6), 1170–1179.

Kidwell, M. C., & Kerig, P. K. (2021). To trust is to survive: Toward a developmental model of moral injury. *Journal of Child & Adolescent Trauma*, 1–17.

King, W. M., Hughto, J. M., & Operario, D. (2020). Transgender stigma: A critical scoping review of definitions, domains, and measures used in empirical research. *Social Science & Medicine, 250*, 112867.

Locke, L. A., & Trolian, T. L. (2018). Microaggressions and social class identity in higher education and student affairs. *New Directions for Student Services, 2018*(162), 63–74.

Masson, J. M. (1985). *The complete letters of Freud to Wilhelm Fliess (1887–1904).* Belknap.

McEwen, C. A., & Gregerson, S. F. (2019). A critical assessment of the adverse childhood experiences study at 20 years. *American Journal of Preventive Medicine, 56*(6), 790–794.

Meyer, I. H. (2003). Prejudice, social stress, and mental health in lesbian, gay, and bisexual populations: Conceptual issues and research evidence. *Psychological Bulletin, 129*(5), 674.

Myers, C. (1915). A contribution to the study of shell shock: Being an account of three cases of loss of memory, vision, smell, and taste, admitted into the Duchess of Westminster's War Hospital, Le Touquet. *The Lancet, 185*(4772), 316–320.

Nadal, K. L. (2018). Measuring LGBTQ microaggressions: The sexual orientation microaggressions scale (SOMS) and the gender identity microaggressions scale (GIMS). *Journal of Homosexuality, 66*(10), 1404–1414.

Nadal, K. L., Griffin, K. E., Wong, Y., Davidoff, K. C., & Davis, L. S. (2017). The injurious relationship between racial microaggressions and physical health: Implications for social work. *Journal of Ethnic & Cultural Diversity in Social Work, 26*(1–2), 6–17.

Nadal, K. L., Griffin, K. E., Wong, Y., Hamit, S., & Rasmus, M. (2014). The impact of racial microaggressions on mental health: Counseling implications for clients of color. *Journal of Counseling & Development, 92*(1), 57–66.

Nemeroff, C. B., Heim, C. M., Thase, M. E., Klein, D. N., Rush, A. J., Schatzberg, A. F., ... Keller, M. B. (2003). Differential responses to psychotherapy versus pharmacotherapy in patients with chronic forms of major depression and childhood trauma. *Focus, 100*(1), 14293–14296.

Pierce, C. (1970). Offensive mechanisms. In C. Pierce & F. B. Barbour (Eds.), *The Black seventies: An extending horizon book* (pp. 265–282). Porter Sargent Publisher.

Redican, E., Nolan, E., Hyland, P., Cloitre, M., McBride, O., Karatzias, T., ... Shevlin, M. (2021). A systematic literature review of factor analytic and mixture models of ICD-11 PTSD and CPTSD using the International Trauma Questionnaire. *Journal of Anxiety Disorders, 79*, 102381.

Resick, P. A., Bovin, M. J., Calloway, A. L., Dick, A. M., King, M. W., Mitchell, K. S., ... Wolf, E. J. (2012). A critical evaluation of the complex PTSD literature: Implications for DSM-5. *Journal of Traumatic Stress, 25*(3), 241–251.

Rich, A. J., Salway, T., Scheim, A., & Poteat, T. (2020). Sexual minority stress theory: Remembering and honoring the work of Virginia Brooks. *LGBT Health, 7*(3), 124–127.

Schmidt, U., & Vermetten, E. (2018). Integrating NIMH research domain criteria (RDoC) into PTSD research. In Vermetten, E., Baker, D. G., & Risbrough, V. B. (Eds.). *Behavioral neurobiology of PTSD* (pp. 69–91). Springer International Publishing.

Schnarrs, P. W., Stone, A. L., Salcido Jr, R., Baldwin, A., Georgiou, C., & Nemeroff, C. B. (2019). Differences in adverse childhood experiences (ACEs) and quality of physical and mental health between transgender and cisgender sexual minorities. *Journal of Psychiatric Research, 119*, 1–6.

Smidt, A. M., & Freyd, J. J. (2018). Government-mandated institutional betrayal. *Journal of Trauma & Dissociation, 19*(5), 491–499.

Struck, S., Stewart-Tufescu, A., Asmundson, A. J., Asmundson, G. G., & Afifi, T. O. (2021). Adverse childhood experiences (ACEs) research: A bibliometric analysis of publication trends over the first 20 years. *Child Abuse & Neglect, 112*, 104895.

Sue, D. W., Capodilupo, C. M., Torino, G. C., Bucceri, J. M., Holder, A., Nadal, K. L., & Esquilin, M. (2007). Racial microaggressions in everyday life: Implications for clinical practice. *American Psychologist, 62*(4), 271.

Valentine, S. E., & Shipherd, J. C. (2018). A systematic review of social stress and mental health among transgender and gender non-conforming people in the United States. *Clinical Psychology Review, 66*, 24–38.

Van der Hart, O., & Horst, R. (1989). The dissociation theory of Pierre Janet. *Journal of Traumatic Stress, 2*(4), 397–412.

van der Kolk, B. A., Pynoos, R. S., Cicchetti, D., Cloitre, M., D'Andrea, W., Ford, J. D., & Teicher, M. (2009). Proposal to include a developmental trauma disorder diagnosis for children and adolescents in DSM-V. *Unpublished manuscript. Verfügbar unter:* http://www. cathymalchiodi. com/dtd_nctsn. pdf (Zugriff: 20.5. 2011).

Wade Jr, R., Cronholm, P. F., Fein, J. A., Forke, C. M., Davis, M. B., Harkins-Schwarz, M., … Bair-Merritt, M. H. (2016). Household and community-level adverse childhood experiences and adult health outcomes in a diverse urban population. *Child Abuse & Neglect, 52,* 135–145.

World Health Organization. (2018). *Adverse childhood experiences international questionnaire.* WHO.

World Health Organization. (2019). *International statistical classification of diseases and related health problems* (11th edition). WHO. https://icd.who.int/

CHAPTER 3

INTERSECTIONALITY 101

The word intersectionality was introduced in a contemporary setting in 1989, by law professor Kimberlé Crenshaw, as a legal term arguing for the recognition of Black cisgender women as a protected class in the context of employment discrimination (1989). At the time, there was no codified legal recognition that a Black cisgender woman might have potentially very different experiences of workplace harassment than either a white cisgender woman or a Black cisgender man, with these different experiences a manifestation of the conjoint systems of white supremacy and patriarchy. Thus, the differential impact of workplace discrimination on Black cisgender women relative to Black cisgender men or white cisgender women was unaccounted for.

Crenshaw acknowledges that the concept described by the term intersectionality predates her work, and that her work grew out of earlier legal work around critical race theory. Over time, the term intersectionality has grown in popularity, especially among Millennials and Zoomers, and use of the word has expanded dramatically in the past decade or so. As intersections of identity in addition to race and gender have been explored and discussed, and discussions of race and gender have expanded to races other than Black and white and genders other than cisgender woman and cisgender man, definitions and usage have continued to grow. It is possible that the way in which the term is used has changed significantly since this writing, so I want to be explicit and clear about what is meant by the term in this particular manuscript, and acknowledge that this may differ from Crenshaw's original intent. Moreover, the word intersectionality and the term critical race theory have been used as bludgeons by the reactionary right, who use these to express something very different than is meant in this manuscript. So, for the sake of clarity, in this manuscript, I use the term intersectional identity, or intersectionality, to describe value-neutral differences in bodies or experiences that come together in an individual and are assessed as "good" or "bad" at the social level. These social assessments, which are rooted in systems that facilitate the development of some individuals and hinder the development of others, are frequently unacknowledged and yet have tremendous impact on people's lives.

Here's an example of what I mean by this. Let's consider an eight-year-old person for a moment. Being eight years old is not an innately good thing or bad thing. In contemporary American society, this individual would be considered a child, although in other parts of the word, and in other historical moments, an eight-year-old might be working in a factory, managing a farm, or married (or all three). Childhood in contemporary American society has a strong connotation of being protected and cared for, but we know at the meta-level of society that voters and politicians (none of whom are children) consistently deprioritize the needs of children, even though investments in children are among the most powerful we can make as a society. So, while being eight years old is neither intrinsically good nor intrinsically bad, this particular aspect of identity has social meaning that can be facilitative (children should be protected) or injurious (as long as it doesn't raise my taxes) to development. Additionally, the identity of being eight years old does not exist in a vacuum. Any particular eight-year-old also has a racial and ethnic identification, a socioeconomic status, a birth-assigned sex and experienced gender, a nascent sexual identity, an ability status, a citizenship and documentation status, a religious identity, and a variety of other identities that

DOI: 10.4324/9781003140740-4

intersect in that individual (hence the term intersectionality). The protection a child is afforded in this country varies greatly as a function of white supremacy (Black children in particular are frequently seen as dangerous by their teachers, for instance; see Young et al., 2018, for a meta-analytic review). Access to protection also varies greatly as a function of capitalism (more than 1.2 million children under the age of six experienced housing instability in the United States in 2018–2019, and unhoused people are far less protected than people with homes; Yamashiro & McLaughlin, 2021). This protection also varies as a function of patriarchy and cisheteronormativity (AFAB children are more likely to experience sexual violence, AMAB children are more likely to experience physical violence, and gender diverse and sexual minority children are at higher risk of all types of violence; these studies will be reviewed in Chapter 4). This protection also varies as a function of ableism (disabled children are at extremely high risk of abuse and neglect; for an overview focused on sexual abuse in individuals with intellectual disabilities, see Byrne, 2018). This protection also varies as a function of social beliefs about body size (fat children are perceived as less worthy of protection, see Morales et al., 2019) and color (darker-skinned children are perceived as less worthy of protection). Thus, the experiences of a queer, AMAB, abled, documented, dark-skinned, thin, Latinx child in a wealthy Midwestern family system will be different than the experience of a straight, cis, AFAB, fat, disabled, undocumented Hmong immigrant in a poor family system on the East Coast. The same systems of oppression will be impacting both of these children, but the ways in which the systems impact these children are mediated by social perceptions of, and beliefs about, the child's intersectional identity.

You may be wondering why I talk about experiences related to intersectional identity as a function of systems such as white supremacy and cisheteronormativity. Although it can seem as if the experiences are different *because* of the ways in which intersections of identity manifest in an individual (for instance, this child couldn't go to a local school *because* she's in a wheelchair), that framing locates the accountability for these experiences in the individual rather than the system. There is nothing intrinsic to using a wheelchair for mobility that keeps someone from attending a particular school. A person in a wheelchair might be prohibited from attending a particular school *because the educational system is ableist*, but it's the ableism that hinders the development of some and facilitates the development of others, not any individual's assistive-device needs. To the extent possible, then, in this manuscript I prefer to use a language of accountability that locates the disparities related to intersectional identity in systems of oppression.

I want to acknowledge from the start that I will make some errors and overlook some forms of systemic oppression in this chapter and in this manuscript. I am certain that there are times in which I slip into ableist language, center white experiences, or speak from a presumption of cisheteronormativity. While it is not your responsibility to bring these lapses to my attention, please know that I welcome your insight if you choose to share it, particularly as it relates to these errors and oversights. It is my intention to be accountable to you and to endeavor to avoid defensive maneuvering when offered feedback that can improve my capacity for accountability.

As conversations about intersectionality have become more frequent in psychological circles, one thing that I have noticed is that sometimes people will say they have "less intersectionality" or "fewer intersections." What I believe people are typically trying to convey when they say they have "less intersectionality" is that they hold several privileged identities, and this generally coincides with having fewer oppressed identities. A white person may feel they do not have a racial identity, for instance, and thus might not recognize the ways in which their whiteness intersects with, say, their working-class socioeconomic status.

Nonetheless, that person does indeed have a racial identity, and exists at the intersection of their white racial identity and their working-class socioeconomic status. This is important because when we say that we have "fewer intersections," this implicitly centers privileged experiences by suggesting that those privileged experiences are "normal" and thus do not contribute to our social location. But privileged identities contribute greatly to our social location. We simply have the opportunity to never necessarily be asked to think about our privileged identities because our survival does not depend on our efforts to understand the experiences of others in those domains in which we are privileged, while it does in those domains in which we are oppressed. For instance, a heterosexual may never have to understand how gay men flirt, but a gay man's survival may well depend on his ability to read the cues of a heterosexual cisgender man. Thus, while heterosexual men do not have to be keen observers of gay flirtation, gay men do have to understand the context of heterosexual mating rituals for their own safety.

The work of exploring intersectionality, at least for clinicians, begins with decentering our own experience by acknowledging our areas of privilege, rather than assuming these areas of privilege are invisible, typical, or innately desirable. A common place for clinicians to start examining our own intersections, and thinking through the cultural biases we hold, is in the ADDRESSING framework (Hays, 1996). The ADDRESSING model is an acronym through which Hays encourages us to consider Age and generation, Developmental disability, Disability acquired later in life, Religion, Ethnicity and race, Socioeconomic status, Sexual identity, National origin and language, and Gender. All of the aforementioned intersect with gender diversity in important ways, which we will begin discussing below. These are also not the only identities we hold that interact with oppressive systems, of course, but I hope this will make a good start for understanding ourselves in relation to our clients and in relation to those systems.

Understanding our own intersectionality is crucial to our work as clinicians because we bring our intersecting identities to the therapy space. Our development has been hindered and facilitated in different ways and at different times by different systems of oppression, just as our clients' development has been. While our focus in therapy is on understanding the experience of the client, this understanding is inevitably constrained by the lens through which we view the world. It is possible to expand the lens, but first we have to acknowledge that the lens exists, and develop a sense of its shape and size.

This is the value of the ADDRESSING framework: it doesn't ask us to consider every possible permutation of intersectional identity we might see in a client in the course of our careers. Instead, it asks us to do some perspective-taking about our own experiences and explore ways in which our unexamined biases might be contributing to systemic oppression in the context of the therapy space. More broadly, we can come to understand the places in which we carry power due to various elements of our identities and learn to recognize the ways in which this socially sanctioned power influences how we see our clients and the judgments we make about them. We can use our understanding of ourselves, then, to guide the hypotheses we create about our clients, and use careful questions about ourselves to test these hypotheses. And, most of all, we can use this incremental advancement in self-awareness, and our understanding of where we are located within power hierarchies, to not get defensive when our clients bump up against our white supremacy, colorism, misogyny, cisheteronormativity, or class-based judgments.

I focus on power and specifically on centering the places in which we are powerful because I know from personal experience how easy it can be to get entrenched in identifying with the places in which we have less power. I remember, for instance, walking down the street on a cold day in Chicago and making eye-contact with someone who I believe was a middle-class, Black, cisgender woman. We smiled at each other and I said, "How're you doing?" but I had only recently moved to Chicago from New York City, and I'm sure what emerged from my mouth was just a whir of sound by Midwestern standards. Her face went from friendly to upset and angry, and I felt myself grow defensive and exasperated. When people see me in passing, they often assume that I am a cisgender man. When they hear my voice, they often get confused about my gender, and sometimes this confusion turns to anger. I assumed that this was what was happening for this woman, so when she didn't respond to my query I shrugged and continued walking. As I passed by, I heard her say, "How dare you? I don't need your change." In that interaction, I had assumed I was experiencing a gender-based microaggression, not realizing that I was participating in a race-based micro-aggression. This woman had assumed that she was experiencing a race-based microaggression, not realizing she was participating in a gender-based microaggression. That both of these microaggressions were based on misperception did not make them any less impactful or painful. Because I am accustomed to gender-based microaggressions as a function of cisheteronormativity, I was not mindful in that moment of my whiteness and white privilege, and how a race-based microaggression as a function of white supremacy might have been playing out for her. Thus, we both missed the opportunity to experience the moment as it was unfolding and instead got stuck in an enactment that was based on our beliefs and past experiences. And while, in this instance, it wasn't the direct responsibility of either of us to move us out of this quagmire, in therapy it *is* the clinician's responsibility to note these enactments and do our level best to move the relationship out of them. We are not able to do that if we are in a space of being self-protective, defensive, or simply low in awareness about our social location.

Let's start by acknowledging that the majority of mental health providers in the United States are white, abled, cisgender women (see Lin et al., 2018, which only allows for a binary representation of gender and does not ask about sexual identity). Because of the educational demands for licensure as a mental health professional, virtually every mental health provider holds educational privilege in comparison with most of our clients, and we often hold socioeconomic privilege as well. This is true even for those of us whose backgrounds involve less educational and socioeconomic privilege than we hold by the time we have achieved our professional status. Moreover, we hold power by virtue of our role as a provider, and this power is separate from, but related to, our other aspects of identity. Finally, there is a very specific role for mental health service providers whose clients are in the pursuit of gender-affirming care, in that sometimes we have literal authority to decide who should be allowed to access specific types of treatment. Notably, nearly every gender-affirming surgery requires a letter of support from a mental health services provider. In some states, and for some people, a letter from a mental health services provider is also required for hormone therapy. This is an awful lot of power vested in the clinician, and if we aren't intentional about addressing it, it can set up a terrible dynamic in which our clients are compelled to be guarded with us, and we feel compelled to "catch" them not being forthright with us or act as gatekeepers "protecting" them from themselves.

I want to be explicit about this power because, as mentioned above, it is much easier to align with the places in which we feel less powerful and to disavow the structural power we do hold. But when we disavow our structural power, we are risking the unwitting participation in acts of aggression toward our clients. Despite internal tension around my experiences with health care providers as a patient, and my own experiences as a health care provider with patients, I do believe that the majority of us have good intentions toward our clients and do not want to aggress against them. So please consider this chapter an invitation to self-reflection and give yourself a chance to think honestly and non-defensively about the stumbling blocks you might encounter as a power-holder in the lives of TGD people who have been exposed to trauma and stress.

I want to now briefly consider each of the ADDRESSING topics as it relates to cis-normativity and TGD experiences. At the end of each section, I invite you to reflect on the ways your relationship with power as experienced through this aspect of your identity may be showing up in your work with clients. I also disclose some elements of my own identity as well as a bit about my current understanding of these elements of my identity vis-à-vis systems of oppression. I offer you some information about my identities for two reasons. First, talking about our identities is hard. Many of us became clinicians so that we could reflect on the identities of others, and it's difficult and often uncomfortable to shift that frame. Because it is something I'm asking you to do, I want to demonstrate a willingness to join you there. Second, we'll be getting into some case studies in later chapters, and I aim to be explicit about identity and power in my formulations, so you will need some information about me for this to make sense in context.

A SHOUT OUT TO THE 2015 USTS

A lot of what we know about the experiences of TGD adults in the United States comes from the 2015 United States Transgender Survey conducted by the National Center for Transgender Equality (NCTE) so you will see this survey referenced many times in this chapter and throughout the rest of this book (James et al., 2016). The 2015 USTS collected data from more than 27,000 TGD adults in the United States (and Americans living abroad) and many of the data-driven studies of TGD experiences are secondary analyses of these data. The TGD community and researchers focused on TGD health have greatly benefitted from the information obtained by the NCTE, and the organization recently announced the launch of another comprehensive survey, with data collection to begin in 2022. Any reference you see to the 2015 USTS in this manuscript is referring to the James et al. document unless otherwise explicitly stated.

AGE AND GENERATION

Because there are TGD people of all ages and all generations, there are some generational differences to bear in mind when working with TGD clients. Over the past decade, the age at which TGD people have typically "come out" as TGD has gotten lower, and with each new generation, the percentage of the population of that generation which identifies as TGD has gotten higher. A 2017 study of generational differences in the LGBT+ community indicates that, while 97% of Boomers and older Gen X identify as cisgender, 94% of younger Gen X and 88% of Millennials identify as cisgender (Gates, 2017). Although this could suggest any number of trends in the data, my interpretation is that it is getting easier for TGD people to come out and live openly in our affirmed genders and that systems such as families and schools are becoming more gender-inclusive and affirming. Additionally, gender-affirming medicine, and especially gender-affirming medicine for children, has become somewhat more accessible, although this is again in flux (and has always been impacted by various forms of structural oppression). Finally, gender identities that are not on the binary are being asked about in research, and more TGD people who do not identify on the binary are using trans as an umbrella term that includes their gender identity or identities. All of these are likely contributing to the observed differences in base rates of TGD individuals across generations.

When working with older TGD clients, especially the Silent Generation and Boomers, but also older Gen X, it is my experience that I observe greater shame and internalized anti-trans bias than I observe in Millennials and Zoomers. Older clients tend to have a later-in-life coming out, more frequently identify on the binary, and tend to have blending as a stronger value than younger people. Thus, there is a stronger tendency toward utilizing the full range of medical transition options available, sometimes coupled with a deep mourning for "lost time" living in the gender associated with their birth-assigned sex. In my experience it is less common for people of these generations to use they/them, or neologisms such as per/pers, as pronouns, and more common to use she/her or he/him. This is probably, at least in part because accessing transition-related medical services used to be even more difficult than it is today, and largely depended on convincing a team of providers in a gender clinic that you were *really* trans (or obtaining treatment through informal and unregulated networks), and some older TGD people have internalized this commitment to the binary. For a review on working with TGD older adults, see Porter et al. (2016).

Gen X and older Millennials tend to be more varied in gender identity and expression than Boomers and the Silent Generation, with some TGD individuals of these generations identifying strongly with the gender binary and others rejecting binary formulations of gender identity and expression. While there was expanding access to options for hormone treatment and gender-affirming surgeries in the 1990s and early 2000s (for affluent, mostly white, Americans in larger and more liberal coastal cities) this medicine continued to be rooted in a binary formulation of gender identity and expression, and hormone dosages, for instance, were not tailored to the individual's goals for their own bodies. I sometimes find that, when working with younger Gen X and older Millennial people who began using HRT when they were young adults, they express a yearning for the options for flexible medicine that are somewhat more available to TGD people beginning medical transition today.

Younger Millennials (and now Zoomers) tend to have more flexible ideas about what gender might be, are more comfortable asking about and sharing pronouns (and less likely to use she/her or he/him), and are more likely to have very specific gender identifications. One part of the historical context here is that TGD Zoomers and younger Millennials is that the internet has always existed in their lifetimes. For those who have access to it, the internet has been a way that individuals have found information about gender-affirming medicine and clinicians, as well as a source of community and support for rural people, people who do not feel safe or comfortable coming out, and members of multiply marginalized communities. And, of course, access isn't equal for all Zoomers and younger Millennials, as internet access and internet literacy differ as a function of socioeconomic status, religious background, and community norms.

I want to take a moment to reflect on TGD elders and TGD children, both of whom are institutionally vulnerable as a function of age. TGD elders may find themselves in living situations (such as state nursing facilities or residential treatment facilities) in which it is dangerous to be out, or in which staff chronically and systematically misgender them or use the wrong name for them. There have even been reports of nursing home staff withholding HRT from TGD patients. On average (although certainly not across the board) older people have more medical needs that are unrelated to gender medicine than younger people, which for many older TGD people might mean disclosing their birth-assigned sex to, for instance, an oncologist or rheumatologist for the first time. On the other end of the age spectrum, TGD children can only access gender-affirming medicine through their caregivers and do not have the right to make decisions regarding their own health care or even the style of clothing they wear or how they keep their hair. (And even with family support and resources, medical transition is no longer available to children in every state.) If a young person is able to access hormone blockers at Tanner Stage 2, they may never have to go through a gender dysphoric puberty, but access to blockers is contingent on family or caregiver approval, even before access to a gender clinic and the financial means to afford the blockers. Additionally, there is increased risk in divulging TGD identity for children, as survival-level family support is sometimes withheld after these disclosures. LGBTQ+, and especially TGD, children and adolescents are overrepresented in youth shelters and in foster care and are at increased risk of abuse from workers in the foster care system as well as from other children in foster care.

Take this opportunity to reflect on your age and generation, and how your age and generation have conferred power in your life. If you are reading this, you are probably over the age of 18, which means that you have the power of adulthood. In what ways do you believe your age and generation contribute to your understanding of gender, and especially to your attitudes toward TGD people of all ages?

Myself, I am at the very young end of Generation X, and I have a strong affiliation with the counter-culture vibe of Gen X. This has probably influenced my identification as genderqueer (rather than nonbinary, for instance), as genderqueer tends to be a more overtly political label.

DEVELOPMENTAL DISABILITY

In 2019, 4.3% of children and youth in the United States were categorized as disabled according to the 2019 American Community Survey. The majority were diagnosed with a cognitive disability. There are any number of ways in which developmental disability might intersect with gender identity for TGD people. But since one major example stands out as especially pertinent, I'll spend most of this section focused on the intersection of gender diversity and neurodiversity (specifically, neurodivergence in the form of autism). The data indicate that autistic people are more likely to be TGD than allistic people, and that TGD people are more likely to be autistic than cisgender people. There is a great deal of speculation about why this might be, which is indeed an interesting research question, but it's important to bear in mind that autistic people, TGD people, and autistic TGD people are generally more interested in obtaining the supports they need than they are in finding that exact genetic signature of either neurodiversity or gender diversity (or "curing" gender diversity of neurodiversity).

Clinical work with gender diverse, neurodiverse populations is the topic of the remarkable book *Supporting Transgender Autistic Youth and Adults: A Guide for Professional and Families* (Gratton, 2019). I strongly encourage you to explore this invaluable resource if you intend to provide therapy to TGD clients (because you will be seeing autistic clients) or autistic clients (because you will be seeing TGD clients). As I have grown to better understand autism and the ways in which neurodiversity can show up in TGD people, I have also come to have a clearer sense of the harm I have caused TGD and autistic clients by not holding more space for their neurodivergence.

Facilitating access to "own voices" material for autistic people who might be TGD, and TGD people who might be autistic, can be very helpful for individuals navigating these experiences. From the systemic side, autistic and allistic caregivers of autistic people, including physicians and clinicians, should be prepared to have conversations about gender identity with the autistic people in our lives. We should also be prepared to believe autistic people when they tell us that they are or may be TGD, and not engage in additional gatekeeping around gender expression that is predicated on judgments about neurodiversity.

I am not aware of data suggesting higher rates of TGD experiences among people with other forms of developmental disability. I imagine, in fact, that explicitly TGD experiences are under-documented among people with intellectual disabilities and Down syndrome, not because people with intellectual disability or Down syndrome aren't TGD, but rather because intellectually abled caregivers may overlook or reject those cues. I have also seen no data on rates of gender diversity among children who are Deaf, blind, or otherwise physically disabled. This is a form of ableist erasure and perhaps also a manifestation of the ableist belief that disabled people don't or shouldn't have sex, and thus developing a gender identity and sexual identity are unimportant tasks in their lives.

Take this opportunity to reflect on your developmental ability status, and how your developmental ability status has conferred power in your life. If you are reading this, you probably do not have an intellectual disability, and if you have a learning disability you probably grew up in an environment that asked you to mask your learning disability and work extra hard, perhaps with additional tutoring, to achieve grade level expectations. If you are reading this you may or may not have been born with a physical disability. In what ways do you believe that your developmental disability status contributes to your understanding of gender, and especially to your attitudes toward TGD people of all abilities?

Myself, I am allistic, and I was not formally diagnosed with a developmental disability in childhood. Because of this, I was tracked into classrooms with other abled children and did not spend much time (that I was aware of, at least) with people with developmental disabilities until I was an adult. I also grew up believing I was physically abled, with few friends who were visibly physically disabled as we were growing up together. These experiences can lend themselves to a kind of saviorism around disability and has sometimes elicited in me the desire to gatekeep around gender and sexuality in disabled people. This is an internal red flag for me—anytime I find myself with the pull toward gatekeeping, I stop and attend to understanding the power structures behind that pull before proceeding.

DISABILITY ACQUIRED LATER IN LIFE

According to the Center for Disease Control, 26% of adult Americans are disabled, most commonly with mobility disabilities followed by cognitive disabilities. According to the 2015 USTS, among TGD adults this is 40% (James et al., 2016). The differences in base rates around disability are probably partially a function of medical oppression and socioeconomic disparity. Although the main barrier to medical care for TGD people is the cost of care (James et al., 2016), even TGD people who are insured, or could otherwise afford, comprehensive medical care, express high rates of mistrust in medical professionals.

Many of the intersections of gender and disability acquired later in life are similar to the intersections of gender and developmental disability as described above. Disabled TGD people report not being taken seriously in their gender identity, and sometimes not having access to forms of transition that would enable a more comfortable gender expression because their caregivers withhold this access.

If you are of the belief that you don't see disabled people in your clinical practice, remember that almost everyone who is treated in the psychotherapy office must be diagnosed with a psychological disability in order to access insurance reimbursement for treatment. Disabilities can be psychological or physical, visible or invisible, and have greater or lesser impact on people's lives. In fact, psychological disability has been, and can be, used to deprive TGD people of medical transition. Currently, the Standard of Care guidelines require the psychological disability be "moderately well-controlled" prior to the initiation of HRT or surgery (World Professional Association for Transgender Health, 2011). For some psychologically disabled TGD people, this is the definition of a double-bind. For instance, coming out as TGD to a trusted clinician and having this identity disavowed could potentiate a borderline crisis in someone with borderline personality disorder. This crisis can then be used as justification for withholding gender-related medicine. It is worth noting that many schizophrenic TGD people first disclose their gender in the midst of a psychotic episode, and this tends to be because they are disinhibited due to the psychosis, not because the person is expressing a gender-related delusion (Smith et al., 2019).

Take a moment to reflect on your current disability status. If you are currently abled, and were to become suddenly physically disabled, what would change in your life? Would you be able to continue living in your current housing situation? Could you keep your job? If not, would that impact the care you are able to receive? Would a shift in your ability status impact your capacity to access medication that is important to you? Why or why not?

As for me, I was diagnosed with a disability later in life, and it took quite some time to understand, or even be fully aware of, my internalized ableism. This can impact my clinical work in that I can experience the desire to jump to advocacy and/or disability pride with my clients and must be conscientious about making plenty of room for people to have their own experiences of their own ability statuses.

RELIGION

About 65% of Americans identify as Christian. The Pew Research Center indicates that 63% of Christians (and 84% of white evangelical Christians) in the United States believe that gender is determined exclusively by sex assigned at birth. This study goes on to indicate that 39% of Christians believe that the United States has "gone too far" in accepting transgender people. It should be noted that 40% of Black Protestants believe that the country hasn't gone far enough in accepting transgender people. It is white Christians, not Black church communities, carrying the effect here.

A recent review of the literature related to religion and transprejudice indicates that identifying as religious, or as Christian or Muslim, was associated with more transprejudice, while identification as nonreligious or Jewish was associated with less transprejudice (Campbell et al., 2019). Additionally, religious fundamentalism and literal interpretations of religious texts also predicted transprejudice across all religious affiliations studied.

Religious traditions of many varieties enforce gendered divisions in expectations for their congregants. Sex-based differences in how and where people of different genders (or, more commonly, different birth-assigned sexes) pray are common to at least some of the forms of all five of the "Big 5" religions (Hinduism, Buddhism, Judaism, Islam, and

Christianity). There are differences in the religious roles available to cisgender men and cisgender women, both in terms of authority to serve as religious leaders, and roles they can serve as members of the laity.

I want to at least reference a topic about which I have very little personal understanding because I have seen it becoming more popular in TGD spaces, and especially with younger Millennials and Zoomers, and that is strong identification with metaphysical spiritual practices such a Wicca or paganism. This sometimes shows up as a strong interest in astrology, or a reverence for plant life, or regular use of divining tools such as tarot cards. While these traditions have been a welcome home for many TGD people, some also report frustration or anger about the focus on Goddesses and Gods, or elements of masculine and feminine energies. I'm not sure how to best understand the rapid proliferation of folk magic practices in TGD spaces but it is something I have observed all across the country, and I want to ensure that clinicians who are unfamiliar with metaphysical spirituality or who struggle with metaphysical practices can learn more and, when necessary, interrogate this difficulty in themselves.

So, this might be a good time to take a moment to consider your religious tradition, and the religious tradition of your upbringing. What messages, if any, did you receive about gender in the context of your religious identity? Were there out transgender members of your church, temple, mosque, or synagogue? Were all religious functions in your tradition open to people of all genders? If not, do you know why not? How do you think your religious tradition has impacted your understanding of gender, and particularly your understanding of TGD people? What would be some of the difficulties for you in working with a TGD person with a very different faith background than yours? What about someone who came from the same faith background and was questioning their faith or turning away from their faith as they explored their gender identity, or had a terrible experience in a religious institution that felt like a home to you?

I was raised in an interfaith home with a pastiche of religious traditions. I don't have any active memories of how religious leaders in my communities talked about TGD people, and my guess is that TGD people were simply not talked about in those communities. When working with TGD clients who grew up in evangelical or fundamentalist homes of any denomination, the risk for me can be a temptation to be overtly or covertly dismissive of the positions their religious leaders take regarding gender identity and expression. For instance, I do not believe in heaven or hell, but some of my clients do fervently believe in these, and grapple deeply with what this means about their TGD identities as well as their hopes and fears about the afterlife.

ETHNICITY AND RACE

There is a misconception among white clinicians that white people in the United States are more likely to be TGD than BIPOC people. The data suggest that this incorrect—that BIPOC people are statistically slightly more likely to identify as TGD than white people (Crissman et al., 2017). There is also the belief among white clinicians that BIPOC families are less inclusive of TGD members than white families. This is somewhat supported by the data from the 2015 USTS (James et al., 2016). The overall percentage of respondents who experienced any form of family rejection was 44%. This was within a few percentage points for Black (47%), Latinx (49%), and Asian American/Pacific Island (AAPI: 46%) respondents. Indigenous respondents reported substantially more experience with family rejection behaviors, with 60% of Indigenous respondents reporting at least one rejecting behavior.

Rejection and acceptance are not diametrically opposed, and some families have high levels of rejection and high levels of acceptance. Indeed, 82% of the overall 2015 USTS (James) sample reported one or more gender-affirming reaction from a family member. Among Black respondents this was 79%, among Latinx respondents this was 81%, among AAPI respondents this was 80%, and among Indigenous respondents this was 78%.

Looking outside the family, there are a variety of forms of socially entrenched difference in experience as a function of white supremacy and patriarchy. We'll talk more about assault and other forms of violence in Chapter 4, but one general example is that white people are often significantly more socially protected if they are read as men when they walk through the world, while Black men almost invariably report wrestling with fears about the ways in which police and state violence will be enacted differently on their bodies if they are perceived as Black men rather than Black women. Given the state violence that is unrelentingly aimed at Black bodies, and especially at the bodies of Black men and masculine-spectrum people, this is a real and present danger that clinicians who are not Black men cannot adequately speak to. Those of us who are not Black men or masculine-spectrum people should encourage our clients to speak with other Black men and masculine-spectrum people in their communities about fear and grief related to police violence, as well as strategies for increasing safety. This could be a matter of life or death, and is not to be taken lightly. Those of us who are not Black women or feminine-spectrum should encourage our clients who are Black women or feminine-spectrum people to think about, talk about, and share tips for safety with other Black women and feminine-spectrum people. Of the 140 identified American TGD women and feminine-spectrum people murdered between 2015 and 2020, more than 75% were Black. Black women and feminine-spectrum people are disproportionately assaulted, attacked, and murdered. This is a function of white supremacy, patriarchy, and anti-trans bias at the intersection of Blackness, femininity, and transness.

Most of us hold a variety of racialized biases, whether implicit or explicit, in our understanding of gender. Tropes about what "men" should be like and what "women" should be like vary from culture to culture, and understandings of masculinity and femininity across cultures are often constrained by the white gaze. For instance, white American culture tends to feminize AAPI men, while hypermasculizing Black and Latino men and hypersexualizing AAPI, Black, and Latina women, and erasing Indigenous men and women entirely. White American culture also tends to be rooted in stereotypes of Middle Eastern and Arab cisgender men as terrorists, and Middle Eastern and Arab cisgender women as downtrodden and subservient, while assuming that Middle Eastern and Arab TGD people don't exist.

There is an additional consideration related to, although separate from, perceptions of race and ethnicity, and that is stigma or bias based on skin color. Sometimes called colorism, this is a manifestation of the white supremacist belief that the closer a BIPOC person is to whiteness, the better, or more attractive, or more trustworthy they are. I use the term colorism to include prioritization of lighter skin (for instance, insisting lighter children stay covered in the sun so they don't get "too dark," or someone resisting a serious relationship with a darker partner because they want "pretty babies"). But colorism can describe other practices not specifically related to skin color, such as plastic surgery on the eyelids of East Asian people to create a rounder (whiter) eye shape, or messages about hair length and texture. There are many racialized (and colorized) standards of beauty in LGBT and TGD communities. This is a particular area of intersection as relates to facial plastic surgery, in which BIPOC TGD people may encounter racist and colorist attitudes about what constitutes beauty (see Plemons, 2019, for a thoughtful overview).

Take a moment to reflect on the role that race and ethnicity have played in your life. How do you feel that your racial and ethnic identities have shaped your understanding of your gender identity? How do you understand racial and ethnic differences in expectations for people of different genders? How do you imagine this might play out differently for a Latino man versus a Filipina woman, despite the putative shared experience of a trans identity?

I am a white person and thus was not asked to consider race or grapple in any meaningful way with white supremacy when I was growing up. My whiteness has probably played the largest role in my development of any identity factor, in that in most contexts I was surrounded by other white people, able to readily access white-centered health and beauty supplies, and educated from within a framework that implicitly and explicitly centered whiteness. Most of the TGD people I know are white, and when I go to TGD or LGBTQ health conferences, most of the attendees are white. What this means in my clinical work with other white people is that I can fall into the trap of implicitly centering our shared experience of whiteness in therapy, and of course white supremacy is often unacknowledged (but very salient) when white people are alone together. Thus, I aim to be explicit about thinking and talking about our whiteness in my relationships with white clients, colleagues, and supervisees. What this can mean for me in my work with BIPOC clients is that I've had to work to get comfortable discussing racism and white supremacy as non-defensively and transparently as I can. It has also meant getting more attuned to the ways in which my BIPOC clients take care of me, often very quickly and seamlessly, when we do talk about white supremacy.

SOCIOECONOMIC STATUS

We can't really talk about gender diversity in the United States without talking about poverty, unemployment, and restricted access to educational opportunity. Let's start with access to educational opportunity, which frequently correlates with long-term earning potential (although this is also stratified based on race). We'll talk more about experiences at school in the next chapter, but among the respondents to the 2015 USTS (James), of those who were out as TGD, or were perceived to be TGD, in K-12, 77% reported adverse experiences, related to gender identity or expression, at school.

While educational achievement is one path toward increased earning potential, it is only helpful in this domain if it leads to more lucrative employment than would otherwise be available. Anti-trans bias limits employment opportunities for TGD people, even those who persist in pursuing their educational goals. Respondents to the 2015 USTS reported 15% unemployment, which was three times the national average the year of the survey. It's important to note that this varied substantially by race. Among AAPI and white respondents, unemployment was 10% and 12%, respectively (about one in ten), or double the national average of 5% (about one in twenty). Among Black, Latinx, and Indigenous respondents, unemployment was closer to one in five (20%, 21%, and 23%, respectively), while among Middle Eastern respondents the rate was more like one in three (35%). Additionally, a secondary analysis of the 2015 USTS found that TGD people who were identifiable to others as TGD were more likely to be unemployed, and that women were more likely to be unemployed than men, reflecting both anti-trans bias and a patriarchal view that sees women and feminine-spectrum people as contributing less to the workplace (Leppel, 2021).

Lack of access to educational and workplace opportunities typically results in poverty, and TGD people are more likely to be poor than cisgender people. Almost one in three of the respondents to the 2015 USTS reported living in poverty (29%). Poverty is difficult in its own right, especially in societies, such as ours, without a robust social safety net. Poverty also contributes to stress, and the stress contributes to anxiety and other forms of psychopathology.

When people are barred from the formal economy, many turn to the informal economy to survive. This is true for TGD people, and nearly 20% of respondents to the 2015 USTS reported having ever engaged in sex work, whether for money, food, drugs, or a place to sleep. Sex work is a high-risk occupation, and about three-fourth of 2015 USTS respondents who reported having sex for income also reported intimate partner violence, with almost as many reporting sexual assault.

If sex work speaks to a particular kind of economic vulnerability, the experience of being unhoused speaks to another, and TGD people are also disproportionately unhoused in the United States. In fact, 30% of respondents to the 2015 USTS reported some form of homelessness at some point in their lives, with this number jumping to 74% among those respondents whose families of origin had kicked them out of their family homes, and 55% among people who had ever lost a job due to anti-trans bias. Moreover, shelters, which are already unsafe living environments, are particularly unsafe for TGD people—70% of the 2015 USTS respondents who had stayed in a shelter in the year preceding the survey reported anti-trans mistreatment in the shelter system.

Take a moment to reflect on your socioeconomic status, and the socioeconomic status you grew up with. Is there a big difference between your childhood SES and your current SES? If so, what are some of the structural factors that contributed to this difference? If not, what are some of the structural factors that contributed to this similarity? If you were to lose your current job, do you feel fairly confident that you would be able to find another? Why, or why not? What role does your gender identity and expression play in your beliefs about your employability and financial security? What are your feelings about people who are experiencing, or have experienced, housing instability? How do you think gender identity and expression influence your feelings about people experiencing housing instability? What are your feelings about people who work, or have worked, as sex workers? How do you think gender identity and expression influence your feelings about sex workers?

Myself, I have lived at a variety of class backgrounds. Like many TGD people of my generation, I left high school before graduating; unlike most people who leave high school without graduating I had the opportunity to later return to college and, ultimately, graduate school. While I was aided in this by having a specific kind of intelligence that happens to be valued in my current society, it was largely facilitated by systemic structures, including white supremacy, that have very little to do with me as an individual.

SEXUAL IDENTITY

A recent Gallup poll found that 86.7% of Americans identify as straight or heterosexual. It is interesting to note that sexual identity in the TGD community is almost the inverse of this general statistic: in the 2015 USTS, 15% of the TGD people surveyed identified as straight or heterosexual. The most commonly reported sexual identity in the 2015 USTS was queer (21%), followed by pansexual (18%).

Based on clinical observation and anecdotal evidence, it seems to me that, as words for gender identity proliferate, neologisms for sexual identity are keeping pace. I do see the two as at least partially intertwined—as new gender identities are expressed, words for sexual identities to describe people who are attracted to those gender identities become necessary. The word lesbian, for instance, has historically been used to describe women who are exclusively attracted to other women, but may be an inaccurate (and in some cases offensive) term for a nonbinary or agender individual who is attracted to women. Neologisms for sexual identity that I have encountered include demisexual (exclusively sexually attracted to people one knows very well), androsexual (attracted to men and masculinity, regardless of biology or anatomy), gynesexual (attracted to women and femininity, regardless of biology or anatomy), and skoliosexual (exclusively attracted to TGD people). Although I acknowledge, with great humility, that I do not know all of the terms for sexual identity, it seems to me to be fundamentally positive to have a broader vocabulary for sexual attraction and desire than lesbian, gay, bisexual, or straight.

I should also acknowledge that all of the above indicates an allosexual perspective (i.e., centering the presumption that all humans experience sexual desire). Asexual people (who do not generally experience sexual desire for others), aromantic people (who do not generally desire romantic connection with others), and people who identify as graysexual, grayromantic, or grayscale (comparatively low sexual or romantic desire for other) are also part of the TGD community. Overall, 10% of respondents to the 2015 USTS identified as asexual, and I think it's possible that this number would be higher today (especially if there were more choices listed that centered asexual experiences). An identification as asexual was particularly high among nonbinary people surveyed by the 2015 USTS, with 17% identifying as asexual. Asexuality is simply another part of the spectrum of sexual desire and should not be conflated with immaturity, fear of sex, or construed as a trauma response, although sometimes people choose not to have sex for any or all of these reasons. Of course, we also live in a society that problematizes and stigmatizes the sexual desire of TGD people, and sometimes TGD people who identify as asexual experience an unexpected change in sexual or romantic desire when they have had the chance to unpack internalized anti-trans bias and sometimes in conjunction with HRT. Sexual identity also may not change as a function of changing gender identity, and that's also valid and real.

TGD people who are, or who are believed to be, sexual minorities experience more exposure to stressors and trauma than TGD people who are, or are believed to be, straight. This is a manifestation of heteronormativity and anti-trans bias operating in tandem at the intersection of sexual identity and gender identity. TGD people of all sexual identities also experience rejection by cisgender sexual minorities, who have sometimes shown themselves willing to sacrifice the goals of TGD people in order to advance a narrow agenda of LGB acceptance.

In addition to questions of sexual attraction based on gender, sexual identity can also be constructed around relationship pattern or type. While some TGD people describe themselves as monogamous, other patterns of relationships, such as polyamory and nonmonogamy, seem, from my clinical experience, to be more common in TGD and LGBT than straight spaces. However, the 2015 USTS found that only 2% of respondents reported being in a polyamorous relationship at the time of the survey. This is very different than a national study that suggests that around 10% of people have tried polyamorous relationships. It seems possible to me that this was at least partially due to how the question was framed, in that it asked about current relationships. Roughly half (49%) of the respondents were single when they completed the survey, and it would be interesting to know if those single people were monogamously or nonmonogamously inclined. As clinicians who work with TGD people, we should be mindful that polyamory and nonmonogamy are simply parts of the spectrum of sexuality.

I want to at least touch on kink as a part of sexual identity, even though I am not aware of solid data about rates of kink orientation in TGD communities. However, like gender itself, kink is becoming a larger part of the sexual landscape for many people in this country, partially inspired by mass market books and movies. Roleplay, crossdressing, and other forms of gender-related fantasy in particular may be a part of the sexual landscape for your TGD clients, so it may be helpful to explore any biases or judgments you may have related to kink, especially if you find yourself pulled toward automatically interpreting kinky behavior as pathology.

Take a moment to reflect on your sexual identity. Do you consider yourself straight? Allosexual? Monogamous? These sexual identities confer a particular kind of social acceptance, so check in with yourself about the structural benefits your sexual identity has conferred. Has there been a time in your lifetime in which you would not be able to marry the partner of your choice due to societal biases related to sexual identity? Are there parts of the world in which it would be illegal for you to express your attraction toward people who express the gender you are most attracted to? Would your sense of your sexual identity change if your gender were to change? What if the gender of your primary romantic or sexual partner were to change? In terms of relationship structure, is there a style of relationship that feels intuitively right to you from a moral perspective? How do you navigate this with your partner or partners? Are sex and romance important to you? If not, what would your work look like with someone to whom sex is very important? If so, what would you work look like with someone who is interested in romance but not sex? Are there relationship structures that seem wrong to you? How might these beliefs get in the way of your ability to offer competent care to TGD individuals?

Myself, I use queer to describe my sexual identity as well as my gender identity, and I appreciate the expansiveness of the label in terms of sexual and romantic attraction. Where I have to be careful with my biases and judgments is when my TGD clients feel constrained in their gender expression as a function of the sexual identity of their partner. In those moments I have to remind myself that there are myriad valid reasons to not transition or not come out, and back off of whatever agenda I might have for this client if they existed in a vacuum.

NATIONAL ORIGIN AND LANGUAGE

Just as there are neologisms in English that are intended to describe a more gender-expansive world, more TGD-inclusive vocabularies are being built in other languages as well. This includes the addition of gender-neutral pronouns that may not have existed before, or the popularization of pronouns that were rarely used. Swedish, for instance, introduced the new pronoun "hen," a gender-neutral alternative to "hon" (she) and "han" (he). Languages vary in their approaches to gender, with some (such as Chinese) already using non-gendered words for pronouns and others (such as Spanish) assigning gender to all nouns and generally signifying the gender of the noun through both the article and the terminal vowel.

Spanish, Chinese, Tagalog, and French are the most commonly spoken languages other than English in the United States, and they deal with gender—and gender diversity—in different ways. If you are a bilingual and/or bicultural therapist, getting comfortable with asking people how they manage pronouns and the language of gender in their other language(s) will be a part of your work. For instance, in some LGBTQ Latinx spaces, the word Latinx is widely adopted and used. Generally, Latinx (or Latine) is used to describe groups that potentially contain people of many genders, or to describe a TGD person for whom Latino or Latina would not be correct. I have also heard Filipinx used in this way as well. This is an evolving usage, however, and I have heard some Latinx and Filipinx people of all genders resist this usage, so asking is, per usual, generally better than presuming.

If you are a bilingual and/or bicultural therapist who works with children and families, it might be difficult to find resources for family members who don't speak English. In this case forums like Reddit can be helpful, as there are often people who will assist in translation. I have yet to find a comprehensive site that provides TGD FAQs, that have been vetted for accurate and culturally aware translation, in multiple languages. I would imagine that such a resource exists—if you know of one, please share. I have had the most luck in finding culturally and linguistically specific resources rather than a site that has a resource translated into several language. However, I also always want to be cautious about recommending resources in languages I don't speak or read (e.g., virtually all of them), as I can't personally assess the quality of the translation or the cultural competence as related to either the language or the information regarding TGD people. In these instances, I have found it most helpful to consult with knowledgeable bilingual and bicultural clinicians (and pay them for their time, of course), but this remains a large area for growth and development and I'm sure there are nuances that I'm missing around the need.

While many people in the United States who speak multiple languages are citizens of the United States, many are not. People from other countries come here for all kinds of reasons, including seeking asylum, in order to join family in the country, and for scholastic and research opportunities. Some immigrants have documentation that allows them to work or study legally, some are in a documentation liminal space (e.g., DACA recipients and people awaiting an asylum evaluation), and some are undocumented.

Many TGD people change our names and/or gender markers on some or all of our official documentation, but not all of us who want to are able to. Undocumented respondents to the 2015 USTS without identification that matched their current gender expression reported physical assault at much higher rates (15%) than the sample overall (2%). Of undocumented respondents to the 2015 USTS who reported having ever been held in immigration detention, 23% were physically assaulted and 15% were sexually assaulted by other detainees or detention officers, and 29% were denied access to hormones. In 2014, a report suggested that on any given day, 75 TGD individuals, including many seeking asylum, are being held in immigration detention. The vast majority are women and feminine-spectrum people, many of whom are housed with detainees who are cisgender men, or held in solitary confinement (for an in-depth web-based report on the experiences of TGD people in immigration detention, see Costantini et al., 2014).

Take a moment to reflect on your national origin, citizenship status, and language (or languages). How have your languages influenced the ways in which you can talk about gender? Are there words in all of your languages that reflect your pronouns? Your gender identity and gender expression? Why or why not? What about your immigration status? Are you a citizen? A documented immigrant? An undocumented immigrant? Do you know anyone who has been deported, or spent time in immigration detention? Have you had that experience? If you have had that experience, or know someone who has, were you (or they) housed with others of the same gender? Why or why not?

Myself, I was born in the United States, and no-one involved with the state machinery of immigration has ever questioned my right to live here. It was easy for me to obtain a driver's license, social security card, and passport when I became an adult. It was also comparatively easy for me to change my name, although access to documentation that reflects my preferred gender marker has been elusive. English is the only language I speak with fluency, and it's a language that does not require I gender groups of people. Although it used to implicitly require gendered individual third-person pronouns, this is becoming less true and has gotten significantly less true in my lifetime.

GENDER

Well, we have now talked a lot about the ways in which gender intersects with a wide range of other aspects of identity. Does gender identity intersect with gender identity? I would argue that individual gender identity and expression does indeed intersect with systemic ideas about gender identity and expression, perhaps most visibly through patriarchy and misogyny. Patriarchy and misogyny devalue attributes and identifiers that are coded as feminine, female, or womanly while normalizing and uplifting attributes that are coded as masculine, male, or manly. Women and feminine-spectrum people frequently find that they are taken less seriously than their colleagues who are men and masculine-spectrum, for instance, and we know that women and feminine-spectrum people are consistently paid less for their labor than men and masculine-spectrum people. Jobs that tend to attract women and feminine-spectrum people tend to be less well-paid, and garner less respect, than comparable jobs that attract men and masculine-spectrum people.

This devaluation of women and feminine-spectrum people is visible in how cisheteronormative society treats feminine-spectrum TGD people versus masculine-spectrum TGD people. TGD spaces are themselves not exempt from misogyny and the devaluation of feminine personhood, and, in fact, some masculine-spectrum people attempt to bolster their masculinity through misogyny and transmisogyny. (This term was introduced in *Whipping Girl: A Transsexual Woman on Sexism and the Scapegoating of Femininity* [Serano, 2007], and has become a cornerstone of transfeminist theory.)

Another way in which misogyny and patriarchy holds space in TGD lives is in the implicit valuation placed on masculinity by hormone regulations and surgery costs. While it is by no means easy to obtain prescriptions for HRT, and all forms of bottom surgery are expensive and uncomfortable, it is more difficult to obtain testosterone than estrogen (testosterone is a Schedule III, and in some states Schedule II, controlled substance), and going from a vagina to a penis is about twice as expensive as going from a penis to a vagina.

In this consideration of gender, and especially reflecting on how we gender bodies, I don't want to miss the opportunity to think about endosexism—that is, the assumption that everyone is born with either a penis or a vagina, and that intersex people either don't exist or are extremely rare. Intersex people are not extremely rare, although endosexism (up to and including forced genital surgery in infancy) has contributed to conditions that lead us to believe they are. For many (endosex and intersex) TGD people and (TGD and cisgender; endosex and intersex) professionals in TGD health, there is natural alliance between endosex TGD people and intersex people of all genders. However, the promise of this alliance has not been well-kept in centrist spaces for professionals focused on TGD health. For an overview of some of the pitfalls and problems, see https://www.transadvocate.com/

owning-endosex-privilege-and-supporting-the-intersex-community-wpath-intersex-genital-mutilation-igm-and-sex-variant-bodies_n_18868.htm

Take a moment to reflect on the role gender has played in your life. Are you cisgender, or are you part of the TGD community? Endosex, or intersex? Does your gender identity or expression confer social power and capital? Has this always been true for you? Are you frequently aware of your gender? Why or why not? Are you frequently aware of the genders of the people around you? Why or why not? How do you feel your experiences with gender, cisnormativity, and patriarchy might influence your work with TGD clients?

Myself I am a masculine-of-center genderqueer individual, with complicated relationships to both masculinities and femininities. My gender expression confers some social power and privilege in that patriarchy confers day-to-day power on masculinity. It is somewhat complicated by the fact that my gender expression transgresses the conventional. This can show up in my clinical work in preconceived judgments about very manly men and very womanly women, demanding caution and extra self-reflection when engaged in work with highly binary individuals.

SIZE AND WEIGHT

Although we have come to the end of the ADDRESSING framework, I want to take this opportunity to speak to another important intersection that may have particular relevance to TGD people. Body policing, diet culture, and anti-fat bias are endemic in this country, including in the therapy space, and size is an often-overlooked element of identity in clinical training (Kinavey & Cool, 2019). Because of this, thin clinicians might not be mindful of the ways in which their offices, practices, and interventions normalize and promote diet culture and a thin ideal. Thin cisgender clinicians might also not be informed about anti-fat bias at the intersection of trans identities.

The 2017 Fat Census solicited survey information from more than 6,000 fat people around the world, but primarily (85%) in the United States (see Shackelford, 2018). Of respondents, 23% described their gender as something other than cisgender. (I am not aware, however, of what percentage of TGD people are fat.) The size of TGD people, and the genders of fat people, are policed and controlled in a variety of ways. Most directly, physicians and medical providers may attempt to control gender expression based on body mass index (BMI). The BMI scale has white supremacist origins (Strings, 2019) and has an innate anti-trans bias in that there are separate scales for (presumably cis) men and (presumably cis) woman (for a nuanced examination of how anti-fatness and anti-transness intersect with anti-Blackness, see Harrison, 2021). TGD people seeking gender-affirming surgeries or hormone therapies will typically have their BMIs evaluated based on their birth-assigned sexes. Fat TGD people may be told they must lose weight prior to obtaining gender-affirming surgeries or hormones, and some report being offered gastric bypass surgery in lieu of gender-affirming procedures. There is limited evidence to suggest that BMI is a meaningful predictor of surgical outcomes for gender-affirming surgical procedures (Brownstone et al., 2021; Ives et al., 2019; Stein et al., 2021).

Outside the medical office, gender expression is frequently associated with the distribution of fat, and the distribution of fat is frequently one of the first changes associated with hormone therapy. Thus, TGD people who are unable to access hormones for whatever reason may endeavor to partially control their gender expression through controlling their body fat. Restricting to conform to an "androgynous ideal" or eating more than desired in the hopes of rounding out breasts or hips are strategies that TGD people sometimes use in an effort to match the body type associated with affirmed genders. Children and adolescents may also restrict in attempts to delay the onset of a dysphoric puberty. Additionally, people in fat bodies are misgendered as a function of anti-fat bias (24% of respondents to the 2017 Fat Census reported having been misgendered as a function of anti-fat bias) or sometimes perceived of as genderless, or as if the gender that a fat person is expressing is the gender of fatness (see Luna, 2018, for personal narrative of this experience). Attempts to control fat distribution are not the only reasons TGD people might consume more or less than their energy needs require, of course, and we'll discuss other ways in which food intake might be impacted in Chapter 6.

Take a moment to reflect on your size, your weight, and the words you use to describe your body. What meanings do the words "fat" and "thin" hold for you? Are those words fairly neutral for you, or do they contain value judgments? How do you feel when your body changes shape or size? How do you believe your weight relates to your gender? Have you felt more pressure to police your body shape and size as a function of your gender expression, or less pressure? Have you ever been denied medical treatment as a function of anti-fat bias?

Myself I have spent most of my life between the high end of a "healthy" BMI and the low end of an "overweight" BMI, with some significant fluctuation in both directions around this marker. I have been protected against some anti-fat bias as a function of my gender expression and against some anti-trans bias as a function of my size (including my weight). It is important to me to have an appreciation for all bodies, but above and beyond that it is important to me to operate within a framework of fat justice or fat liberation. But that is not where everyone is, and I have to be careful to remember that people want different things for their bodies. Sometimes the things people want for their bodies are predicated on diet culture and cisheteronormativity, and those things are still what they want.

IN SUM

We have covered a lot of ground in this chapter and still only skimmed the surface regarding concepts of intersectional identity. Learning about ourselves, and understanding our various social locations, is a life-long journey. Wherever you are on that journey, I appreciate your willingness to spend some time on the path with me.

WORKS CITED

Brownstone, L. M., DeRieux, J., Kelly, D. A., Sumlin, L. J., & Gaudiani, J. L. (2021). Body mass index requirements for gender-affirming surgeries are not empirically based. *Transgender Health*, 6(3), 121–124.

Byrne, G. (2018). Prevalence and psychological sequelae of sexual abuse among individuals with an intellectual disability: A review of the recent literature. *Journal of Intellectual Disabilities*, 22(3), 294–310.

Campbell, M., Hinton, J. D. X., & Anderson, J. R. (2019, February 19). A systematic review of the relationship between religion and attitudes toward transgender and gender-variant people. *International Journal of Transgenderism*, 20(1), 21–38. doi:10.1080/15532739.2018.1 545149

Costantini, C., Rivas, J., & Rios, K. (2014). *Why did the US lock up these women with men?* http://interactive.fusion.net/trans/

Crenshaw, K. (1989). Demarginalizing the intersection of race and sex: A black feminist critique of antidiscrimination doctrine, feminist theory and antiracist politics. *The University of Chicago Legal Forum*, 139–167.

Crissman, H. P., Berger, M. B., Graham, L. F., & Dalton, V. K. (2017). Transgender demographics: A household probability sample of US adults, 2014. *American Journal of Public Health, 107*(2), 213–215.

Gates, G. J. (2017). LGBT data collection amid social and demographic shifts of the US LGBT community. *American Journal of Public Health, 107*(8), 1220–1222.

Gratton, F. V. (2019). *Supporting transgender autistic youth and adults: A guide for professionals and families.* Jessica Kingsley Publishers.

Harrison, D. L. (2021). *Belly of the Beast: The Politics of Anti-Fatness as Anti-Blackness.* North Atlantic Books.

Hays, P. A. (1996). Addressing the complexities of culture and gender in counseling. *Journal of Counseling & Development, 74*(4), 332–338.

Ives, G. C., Fein, L. A., Finch, L., Sluiter, E. C., Lane, M., Kuzon, W. M., & Salgado, C. J. (2019). Evaluation of BMI as a risk factor for complications following gender-affirming penile inversion vaginoplasty. *Plastic and Reconstructive Surgery Global Open, 7*(3), e2097.

James, S. E., Herman, J. L., Rankin, S., Keisling, M., Mottet, L., & Anafi, M. (2016). *The report of the 2015 U.S. transgender survey.* National Center for Transgender Equality.

Kinavey, H., & Cool, C. (2019). The broken lens: How anti-fat bias in psychotherapy is harming our clients and what to do about it. *Women & Therapy, 42*(1–2), 116–130.

Leppel, K. (2021). Transgender men and women in 2015: Employed, unemployed, or not in the labor force. *Journal of Homosexuality, 68*(2), 203–229.

Lin, L., Stamm, K., & Christidis, P. (2018). *Demographics of the US psychology workforce: Findings from the 2007–16 American community survey.* American Psychological Association Center for Workforce Studies.

Luna, C. (2018). *The gender non-conformity of my fatness.* The Body Is Not an Apology. https://thebodyisnotanapology.com/magazine/the-gender-nonconformity-of-my-fatness

Morales, D. X., Grineski, S. E., & Collins, T. W. (2019). School bullying, body size, and gender: An intersectionality approach to understanding US children's bullying victimization. *British Journal of Sociology of Education, 40*(8), 1121–1137.

Plemons, E. (2019). Gender, ethnicity, and transgender embodiment: Interrogating classification in facial feminization surgery. *Body & Society, 25*(1), 3–28.

Porter, K. E., Brennan-Ing, M., Chang, S. C., Dickey, L. M., Singh, A. A., Bower, K. L., & Witten, T. M. (2016). Providing competent and affirming services for transgender and gender nonconforming older adults. *Clinical Gerontologist, 39*(5), 366–388.

Serano, J. (2007). *Whipping girl: A transsexual woman on sexism and the scapegoating of femininity.* Seal Press.

Shackelford, H. A. (2018). *The executive summary of the 2017 Fat Census.* Free Figure Revolution.

Smith, W. B., Goldhammer, H., & Keuroghlian, A. S. (2019). Affirming gender identity of patients with serious mental illness. *Psychiatry Online.* https://doi.org/10.1176/appi.ps.201800232

Stein, M. J., Grigor, E., Hardy, J., & Jarmuske, M. (2021). Surgical and patient-reported outcomes following double incision and free nipple grafting for female to male gender affirmation: Does obesity make a difference? *Journal of Plastic, Reconstructive & Aesthetic Surgery, 74*(8), 1743–1751.

Strings, S. (2019). *Fearing the black body.* New York University Press.

World Professional Association for Transgender Health. (2011, September). *Standards of care for the health of transsexual, transgender, and gender nonconforming people, seventh version.* http://www. wpath.org/publications_standards.cfm. Accessed April 10, 2012.

Yamashiro, A., & McLaughlin, J. (2021). *Early childhood homelessness state profiles: Data collected in 2018–19.* Office of Planning, Evaluation and Policy Development, US Department of Education.

Young, J. L., Young, J. R., & Butler, B. R. (2018). A student saved is NOT a dollar earned: A meta-analysis of school disparities in discipline practice toward Black children. *Taboo: The Journal of Culture and Education, 17*(4), 6.

CHAPTER 4

TRAUMATIC AND STRESSFUL EXPERIENCES IN THE LIVES OF TRANS PEOPLE

Transgender and gender diverse people are at high risk, at the population level, of exposure to the variety of stressors discussed in Chapter 2. While this chapter outlines some of the literature specifically related to trauma and stress exposure in TGD populations, I want to preface the chapter with a reminder that different TGD people in different TGD communities are differentially impacted by these stressors. As discussed in Chapter 3, some TGD people have more protection from trauma and stress than others, while some are at greatly increased risk of exposure. Moreover, some TGD people are embedded in family systems or community systems that provide the support that can buffer against developing PTSD or CPTSD in the wake of trauma exposure, while others are embedded in family systems or community systems that perpetuate harm (and most have both protective and destructive people and systems in their lives). That said, I personally have not encountered a TGD person who reports having absolutely no experience with anti-trans bias. While I may have known some TGD people who have never experienced anti-trans physical violence, I do not know any TGD people who have never worried about anti-trans physical violence nor do I know any TGD people who have never modified their choices around gender expression out of fear of encountering anti-trans violence. I do recognize, however, that my anecdotal experiences are not data that could be construed as representative of population-level data. Thus, this chapter focuses primarily on research that reveals trends in the available TGD data and, where the research base is sparse, presents information or context drawn from clinical experience. Moreover, in the second half of the chapter, we'll move into data that are entirely clinical, introducing the case studies that will be followed for the rest of the manuscript.

TGD PEOPLE AND CRITERION A STRESSORS

According to the 2015 United States Transgender Survey (James et al., 2016), 9% of TGD survey respondents were physically attacked as a function of anti-trans bias in the year prior to participating in the survey. While respondents reported attacks attributed to identity markers other than gender expression (notably sexual orientation), physical attack as a function of anti-trans bias was by far more common than physical attack ascribed to other biases. Moreover, people in some TGD communities reported much higher rates of physical attack in the year prior to the survey than others. For instance, 41% of respondents who were working in the informal economy in that year reported having been physically attacked, as did 24% of undocumented respondents. Middle Eastern (25%) and Indigenous (25%) respondents also reported elevated rates of physical attack. Those respondents who reported having been physically attacked in the last year were also asked how many physical attacks they had experienced. In this survey, 45% of those respondents who had been physically attacked in the year prior to the survey reported one physical attack in that year, while 16% reported four or more attacks.

Turning to other sources of data, a recent study of women living in the San Francisco Bay Area stratified risk of exposure to hate crimes based on the participant's race and ethnicity and also based on how frequently each woman's gender was questioned by others

DOI: 10.4324/9781003140740-5

(Gyamerah et al., 2021). This study found that Latina and Black women were more likely to have experienced battery with a weapon than white women and women of other races. The white women and women of other races in this study reported more exposure to transphobic sexual assault than the Black and Latina women. An earlier study of 97 women and feminine-spectrum people examined the frequency of potentially traumatizing events in the lives of participants using the Traumatic Life Events Questionnaire (Shipherd et al., 2011). Almost all (98%) of the respondents reported at least one potentially traumatizing event, and 91% endorsed multiple traumatizing events. Among those participants who had experienced potentially traumatizing events, slightly fewer than half (46%) reported that at least one of the potentially traumatizing life events was a function of anti-trans bias. Of the 28 participants who had been hit or badly beaten by a stranger, 13 of these reported that this had been a function of anti-trans bias.

An overview of violence in TGD communities consolidated data from multiple sources, including journal articles, social services records, and police reports (Stotzer, 2009). In addition to providing a discussion of the pros and cons of each source (including the acknowledgment that many of these acts of violence go unreported for a variety of reasons), this overview reiterated that rates of anti-trans violence are high, and that members of some TGD communities—most especially sex workers—are at higher risk of violence than members of other TGD communities. This article also makes the point that violence against TGD people is not taking place as one-off events, but rather that TGD survivors of anti-trans violence are victimized across the lifespan and experience multiple forms of victimization. Another review of studies regarding violence related to sexual and gender identity found that the prevalence of violence exposure in TGD respondents to these studies varied from 11.8% to 68.2%, further underscoring the variation that exists from sample to sample (Blondeel et al., 2018).

In addition to experiencing increased risk of physical violence from strangers, TGD people are also at increased risk of intimate partner violence (IPV). Among those respondents to the 2015 USTS (James) who had ever had an intimate partner, 54% reported IPV of any kind, 35% reported physical IPV, and 24% reported severe IPV. Again, this risk was stratified by other identity factors. Past and current sex workers (77%) and previously and currently unhoused respondents (72%) experienced the most elevated risk, with disabled people and undocumented people also reporting high exposure to IPV. When stratified by race and ethnicity, Indigenous respondents reported the highest levels of IPV (73%) and AAPI respondents the lowest (43%). The percentages change somewhat, but the patterns hold steady, when looking at physical IPV exclusively: TGD people are at high risk of physical IPV, and this risk is concentrated among TGD people with multiple marginalized identities. Not all IPV against TGD people is predicated on anti-trans bias, but rather TGD status confers an additional level of risk of experiencing violence, including IPV.

In addition to physical violence, TGD people experience elevated risk of sexual assault. In the 2015 USTS, 10% of respondents reported having been sexually assaulted in the year prior to taking the survey, and when looking at lifetime sexual assault rates, almost half (47%) of the respondents reported having been sexually assaulted in their lifetime. Experiences of sexual assault were most reported by people who were or had been sex workers (72%), were or had been unhoused (65%) and disabled people (61%). Sexual assault experiences were also higher in communities of color, with Indigenous (65%) and multiracial (59%) respondents reporting the highest rates of lifetime sexual assault. There were also differences in the experience of sexual assault based on sex assigned at birth, with AFAB respondents reporting higher rates of lifetime sexual assault than AMAB individuals. Among those respondents who reported sexual assault, most reported having been assaulted by a friend (47%) or by a partner or ex-partner (34%).

Although it seems likely that many of these studies are primarily focused on exposure to violence that would meet Criterion A thresholds for PTSD, it is difficult to fully assess because, unless a study is specifically focused on the PTSD diagnostic criteria, questions about trauma exposure are not typically framed to assess for this information. Additionally, as examined in a recent study of TGD people with PTSD, stressors that would not meet Criterion A, such as anti-TGD bias and non-affirmation of gender, contribute to PTSD symptom severity in TGD people with PTSD, with internalized transphobia playing a mediating role (Barr et al., 2021). This relationship was consistent even when controlling for Criterion A stressors. Thus, focusing on Criterion A stressors alone would leave us with a diminished understanding of the diagnostic impact of other types of stressors. This study built on a study of discriminatory experiences in a TGD sample, which found that even after controlling for exposure to Criterion A stressors, PTSD symptom severity was predicted by more experience with everyday discrimination, including being treated with less courtesy than others (Reisner et al., 2016).

We turn now to some other types of stressors, starting with adverse childhood experiences (ACEs). As we do, please bear in mind that some ACEs *would* meet the threshold for Criterion A, and also that distinguishing between types of trauma and the sequelae of types of trauma is not a clear-cut proposition.

TGD PEOPLE AND ACES

There is a body of literature to suggest that cisgender sexual minorities are at increased risk of ACEs relative to cisgender straight people, and that health disparities can be at least partially attributed to these differences in ACEs (see, for instance, Austin et al., 2016). One recent study of LGBTQ+ individuals indicates that 40% of LGBTQ+ people report three or more ACEs, as compared to a national average of 10% (Bond et al., 2021). While the LGB, and sexual and gender minority, literature around ACEs is growing, TGD participants are sometimes either excluded from these studies, or their data is not analyzed separately from the data of cisgender sexual minorities. As mentioned in Chapter 2, however, a recent study does focus on ACEs in TGD people as compared to cisgender sexual minorities (Schnarrs et al., 2019). This study administered the ACEs questionnaire as well as additional questionnaires related to physical and mental health to sexual and gender minorities. Of the 477 participants who completed the study, 21.4% identified as TGD. The vast majority of respondents (86.2%) reported experiencing at least one ACE, while 91.2% of the TGD respondents reported at least one ACE. More than half of all of the participants (53.6%) reported growing up in a home in which there was emotional abuse, and almost half (49%) reported growing up in a home with a psychologically disabled adult. The TGD respondents were more likely to report emotional abuse, and both physical and emotional neglect, than the cisgender sexual minority respondents. Among the TGD respondents, 4.9% reported having experienced all ten ACEs, as compared to 1.1% of the cisgender sexual minority group.

Although not specifically focused on ACEs, but rather utilizing a survey based on ACEs questions, a recent study comparing rates of physical, sexual, and psychological abuse in cisgender and TGD adolescents found that TGD adolescents were at increased risk for each of these forms of abuse (Thoma et al., 2021). When the cisgender group was stratified by sexual identity, the TGD group reported higher rates of psychological, and physical abuse than either the straight cisgender group or the sexual minority cisgender group. When the TGD group was stratified by gender identity, boys and AFAB nonbinary individuals reported higher rates of psychological abuse, and adolescents questioning their gender identity reported higher rates of physical abuse. In terms of sexual abuse, while the TGD group reported higher rates than the cisgender group, when stratified by gender identity the TGD groups did not differ significantly from the cisgender girls.

A recent Letter to the Editor of the *Journal of Gay and Lesbian Mental Health* made the argument that a more robust literature on the effect of ACEs on TGD people particularly is necessary (Kroppman et al., 2021). This letter also made the case that a more expansive list of ACEs might be appropriate for TGD people, and that being forced to wear clothing or participate in activities associated with their birth-assigned sex might be uniquely adverse, and potentially explain some of the health-disparities data, for TGD youth. A review of the literature related to child abuse of TGD people in childhood speaks to the high rates of abuse of TGD people, and of related deleterious effects to physical and mental health (Tobin & Delaney, 2019).

TGD PEOPLE AND MICROAGGRESSIONS

The study of microaggressions has both quantitative and qualitative components, although until fairly recently there was little quantitative research on gender-based microaggressions aimed at TGD people. This was at least in part because there was not a validated measure for reporting microaggressions rooted in anti-trans bias. A recent triad of studies introduced the Gender Identity Microaggressions Scale (GIMS) and added additional validation of the Sexual Orientation Microaggressions Scale (SOMS; Nadal, 2018). Principal components analysis of the GIMS questions described five categories of microaggressions related to gender identity and expression: denial of gender identity, misuse of pronouns, invasion of bodily privacy, behavioral discomfort, and denial of societal transphobia.

From the qualitative literature, it becomes clear that microaggressions reflecting anti-trans bias take place across multiple domains of experience and in the context of multiple types of relationships. An early qualitative study identified 12 themes of microaggressions rooted in anti-trans bias, including systemic and environmental microaggressions, and microaggressions within given family systems (Nadal et al., 2012). A review of the TGD microaggressions literature identifies several areas that were and remain under-researched in this domain, including microaggressions in the family, among friends, and in the workplace (Chang & Chung, 2015). A study that focused on microaggressions in TGD people in the context of friendships, identified nine categories of potential microaggression, including endorsement of the gender binary, use of transphobic language, and tokenization (Galupo et al., 2014). These microaggressions were enacted more frequently by the participants' cisgender friends, including LGBQ+ cisgender friends, but the qualitative portion of the study suggested that the microaggressions were more painful coming from other TGD people. A related manuscript investigates microaggressions experienced by TGD people in the context of romantic relationships through thematic analysis and identifying four relevant themes (Pulice-Farrow et al., 2017). Two of these are at least partially related to gender presentation and social judgment, namely gendered expectations and public negotiation of gender identity. Finally, at least two thematic analyses have focused TGD people's experience of missteps and microaggressions in the context of therapy (Mizock & Lundquist, 2016; Morris et al., 2020). Identifying therapist lack of experience and education regarding TGD people, one of these studies acknowledges that, while frequently unintentional, therapist microaggressions against TGD clients are pervasive and harmful and constitute ethical guideline violations as defined by the American Psychological Association (Morris). The four themes that emerged from this research were lack of respect for client identity, lack of competency, saliency of identity, and gatekeeping. An earlier study provides grounded theory analysis of missteps that therapists make in counseling TGD people, including gender avoidance and education burdening (Mizock). We will revisit these studies in Chapter 9.

TGD PEOPLE AND INSTITUTIONAL BETRAYAL

Institutional betrayal is a concept that refers to ways in which social institutions that are intended to protect individuals in their care compound, or are otherwise complicit in, traumatic events perpetrated by individuals involved in with the institution on another individual involved with the institution (for a broader contextual discussion see Smith & Freyd, 2014). A classic example is when a college student sexually assaults another college student, and the college revictimizes the victim by refusing to take action against the perpetrator (or sometimes taking action against the victim on behalf of the perpetrator). People who are in contexts in which they are highly dependent on a particular system in order to meet their needs (e.g., people in prisons, people in the military, and people seeking medical care) are especially vulnerable to institutional betrayal, whether or not the individual trusts the particular system on which they are dependent. Institutional betrayal can, in theory, take place irrespective of privilege, but in reality people who hold multiple marginalized identities are far more likely to experience various forms of institutional betrayal. For TGD people, institutional betrayal may be salient in many facets of life, but the focus here is on detention facilities (jails, prisons, and immigration detention), the military, schools, religious institutions, and the medical system.

More than half (58%) of respondents to the 2015 USTS who had interacted with a law enforcement officer who know or thought the respondent was TGD in the year prior to the survey reported experiencing at least one form of mistreatment (James). This was significantly higher among unhoused (78%), unemployed (75%), and disabled (68%) as well as Indigenous (74%), multiracial (71%), Latinx (66%), and Black (61%) respondents. Among respondents who had been were incarcerated in the past two years (2%) 30% reported being physically or sexually assaulted by an officer or another inmate in the past year. Rates of incarceration are significantly higher in the undocumented population, and immigration detention has specific risks for TGD people as discussed in Chapter 3.

TGD people are generally housed with inmates of their birth-assigned sex, and those who are taking hormones are frequently prohibited from access to this treatment. TGD people are overrepresented in prisons, jails, juvenile detention, and immigration detention. One recent review focused entirely on research pertaining to incarcerated TGD people, primarily in the United States but with the inclusion of a couple of studies from Australia (Brömdal et al., 2019). This study found themes of increased risk of sexual assault among TGD prisoners and also reported themes of coercive sex, the conditions of which were sometimes accepted by the TGD person for protection or security. Unfortunately, sexual relationships in prison are associated with greater risk of violence, sexual maltreatment, and sexual assault for TGD prisoners rather than less risk (Jenness & Sexton, 2021).

In regards to military service, TGD people serve in the military at two to three times the rate of the cisgender population, and the United States Department of Defense is the largest employer in the world. There are a lot of TGD veterans and active service personnel, and the Veteran's Health Administration is the health care entity serving the largest number of TGD people in the country. At the time of this writing, the ban on TGD people serving openly in the US military has been lifted, but this has been very unstable since 2016. (In 2016, a blanket ban on TGD people in the military, which had been in place since 1960, was lifted, but there were several changes to the rules and regulations from 2016 to 2021, and may yet be additional changes ahead.) Because of this, there is limited information about the experiences of TGD people in the military, as many have been reluctant to risk outing themselves to researchers when this could cost them their livelihoods. For a qualitative overview of the research priorities, and barriers to research participation, of TGD military personal, see Wolfe et al. (2021).

Of respondents to the 2015 USTS who had separated from the military, 19% reported separating in order to avoid harassment or mistreatment related to anti-TGD bias. This was higher among Latinx (28%) and Black (26%) respondents. Military sexual assault (MSA) is also a risk for TGD military personnel, with a study of 221 TGD veterans indicating the 17.2% of the overall sample reported MSA, including 30% of the men and 15% of the women (Beckman et al., 2018).

Schools are also institutions with increased risk for TGD people. According to the 2015 USTS, 77% of respondents who were out as TGD (or thought to be TGD) in K-12 education, and 24% of respondents who were out/thought to be TGD in college or vocational school experienced some form of anti-trans discrimination (James). Among respondent who were out/thought to be TGD in K-12, harassment caused 17% to drop out of school. A recent study of 3,673 TGD children and adolescents in middle school and high school found that, in the previous 12-month period, 27% of the AFAB nonbinary participants and 26.5% of the boys were sexually assaulted as well as 17.6% of the girls and 16.5% of the AMAB nonbinary participants (Murchison et al., 2019). Restricted access to bathrooms and locker rooms increased the likelihood of sexual assault at school, especially for the girls in this study. In a study of college students, data collected from 2011 to 2013 indicated that TGD students were more likely to experience sexual victimization, physical victimization, and verbal victimization than their cisgender counterparts (Griner et al., 2020).

In considering institutional betrayal in religious settings, according to the 2015 USTS, the majority (68%) of respondents had been a part of a religious community at some point in their lives, with Black (77%) and Middle Eastern (71%) respondents the most likely to endorse this experience. Of those respondents who had been raised in, or ever been a part of, a religious community, 19% left at least one religious community due to rejection of their TGD identity. There was also an effect of race and ethnicity on this phenomenon, with 33% of Indigenous respondents, and 24% of Black and Middle Eastern respondents, who had been part of a faith community leaving that community due to rejection. Turning to other sources of data, a recent study of religion and spirituality in TGD communities suggests that about half of the sample experienced rejection in religious communities, and that having experienced this rejection was associated with more spiritual and religious struggle (Exline et al., 2021).

As painful and stressful as rejection by a religious community can be, being forced to attempt to conform to cisheteronormativity in order to keep a religious community is also damaging. A recent study that performed secondary analyses on the 2015 USTS data found a relationship between lifetime exposure to conversion therapy and number of lifetime suicide attempts, whether the conversion therapy was performed by a secular or religious professional (Turban et al., 2020).

While conversion therapy is not the only form of institutional betrayal in religious settings, and conversion therapy can also take place in secular settings, I draw attention to it here as a bridge between failures of religious institutions and failures of healthcare institutions, and perhaps especially psychology and psychiatry. Much of the history of psychology and psychiatry as pertains to gender has been to "encourage" TGD people to take greater interest and satisfaction in the pursuits, activities, and modes of dress more typical of the gender associated with the individual's birth-assigned sex. The harms of conversion therapy, as well as a comprehensive outline of a model ban on the practice, is detailed in Ashley, 2022. Conversion therapy is dangerous for sexual and gender minorities: a study of a younger (ages 13–24) cohort of LGBTQ individuals found that the group which had experienced conversion efforts focused on sexual or gender identity was twice as likely to report suicide attempts (Green et al., 2020).

Outside of the risk of conversion therapy, the 2015 USTS found that 33% of respondents who had seen a medical provider in the previous year reported negative experiences with providers, ranging from being asked to educate providers about TGD people to being verbally, physically, or sexually assaulted while seeking medical care. These experiences are partially a function of visibility—a cross-sectional study of people who described themselves as recognizably TGD were more likely to report discrimination or victimization in health care settings than TGD people who described themselves as less recognizably TGD (Rodriguez et al., 2018).

TGD PEOPLE AND MORAL INJURY

This is a difficult section to write because this is a difficult topic to address. As most of us who work with trauma survivors know, the pool of survivors and perpetrators is not separate. In fact, the overlap of the Venn diagram is very large, and sometimes people are both things at once in the same interaction. There is a body of literature of research on trauma history in cisgender perpetrators of violence in straight relationships (see, for instance, Hilton et al., 2019; Miles-McLean et al., 2021; Semiatin et al., 2017). There is a growing body of literature on violence in same-gender relationships (see, e.g., Reuter et al., 2017). There are also recent reviews, one focused on availability of services for LGBTQ perpetrators of IPV (Cannon, 2019) and one literature review of articles related to such services (Subirana-Malaret et al., 2019). But as far as I have been able to find, there is very little that even acknowledges the possibility that TGD people might perpetrate violence, other than the scare-mongering right-wing propaganda that insists TGD people are sexual predators with no evidence to support this insistence. Indeed, I can see why researchers and clinicians would shy away from even asking questions about TGD perpetration, knowing these could easily be used as horrific rationale for further anti-TGD legislation.

That said, as discussed above, TGD people experience high rates of violence, and people who have experienced violence sometimes go on to perpetrate it. As a clinician, it is important to me to be unequivocally on the side of my client. And, sometimes, being fully and radically on someone's side means sitting with them through the horror of acknowledging that they have hurt someone else. Acknowledging the damage that we, as humans, have done to one another is a vital and very difficult step in getting free from this pattern of violence.

While there are many forms of this, there is a specifically TGD-related phenomena that sometimes presents itself in clinical practice, and that is TGD people who have come out who are now looking back at anti-TGD acts of violence they participated in. Sometimes this has taken the form of anti-TGD or anti-LGBTQ+ bullying online and/or in real life. Sometimes it has taken the form of anti-TGD violence. And, of course, we all participate in structural violence against TGD people every day, although some people may be more active than others in this (through voting, hiring practices, etc.) An interesting personal narrative that speaks to the experience of bullying out TGD people prior to coming out is by Evey Winters, and currently available at https://eveywinters.com/genital-preferences-or-bigotry/. While the theme of this essay is genital preference, the discussion about anti-TGD bigotry in people who later identify openly as TGD begins in the section of the essay titled "A True King Doesn't Have to Say It."

INTRODUCING THE CASE HISTORIES

While I have a deep and abiding love of statistical models and manuscripts that center quantitative data, I must acknowledge that I have learned that this is adjunctive for me when it comes to understanding my clients and the ways in which therapy might unfold in the moment-to-moment experience. So, now that this manuscript has established a mutual vocabulary for talking about gender, trauma, and intersectional identity and has presented some data-driven information regarding the lives of TGD people, I want to also add some composite case studies to contextualize these various sources of information. I'll start by acknowledging that each of these three case studies is a composite of numerous people seen over the course of my career. Although I have endeavored to present realistic case studies that capture the profiles of the kinds of clients I have worked with, no case study in this manuscript is based on any one person, and any similarity to any person, living or dead, is purely coincidental.

Advika

When Advika first came to see me, she was dressed in a pink kurta worn over jeans, with a chin-length, layered haircut. They were wearing a number of gold rings on their finger as well as two in their right nostril. In our first session, Advika explained that she was an immigrant from Jaipur, identified as bisexual, and thought she might be a feminine man or a genderfluid trans woman, and wanted me to use she/her and they/them (roughly equally) as pronouns. She was wondering about testosterone suppression and the addition of estrogen, and she wanted to talk through her feelings about these possibilities as well as get a recommendation for a gender-affirming prescriber.

Advika used the name Advika across all contexts in the United States, but used a different name at home in Jaipur and had not changed their name or gender marker on any of their identification. She presented to treatment at a fairly early stage of gender exploration, with gender as the presenting rationale for seeking treatment, but in our initial meeting, it quickly became clear that she was primarily preoccupied with questions related to focus, including feeling checked out and absent much of the time. They mentioned previous treatment in college through the school's counseling center, which they had found helpful.

Advika was an only child of married parents who were both affluent and professionally successful and described a great deal of pressure to live up to those benchmarks. She had immigrated to the United States for college, had gone on to obtain both undergraduate and graduate degree in computer science from a prestigious university on the west coast, and was working for a tech startup, putting in very long days with multiple competing priorities; she described no difficulty with focus while at work. They described a large and involved extended family, and frequently returned to Jaipur for holidays and family weddings, and often felt pulled between workplace expectations and familial obligations. She described her parents as generally supportive of her, while acknowledging that there was pressure from them and other family members for her to conform to expectations of masculinity for the sake of harmony in the family. Specifically, their grandmother wanted them to get married (to a "suitable" cisgender woman) and begin working on the next generation. She had cousins her age and younger who were marrying and having children, and she felt she was fast approaching a decision-point in which she would either have to come out, or commit to life lived passing as a straight, cisgender man. They described feeling this would be unfair to their potential future wife but struggled with the belief that making a different choice would be unfair to their family of origin.

Advika's parents had very time-consuming and demanding jobs when she was growing up, and Advika was largely raised by a nanny until the age of 9, at which point her grandmother moved into the home and became her primary caregiver. This change in caregiving was precipitated by the discovery that Advika had been stealing some of their cousin's clothes, and wearing these purloined "girl clothes" around the house (which their nanny knew, but had never mentioned to other adults in the home). Advika reported feeling a great sense of shame when the theft was discovered as well as grief and confusion about losing her primary caregiver very rapidly and without explanation.

Advika described a childhood that was characterized by a feeling of being on the outside looking in. Although they had cousins and same-age family members in their life, they found it difficult to connect and also described emotional neglect from their parents, and some emotional and physical maltreatment from their grandmother when she became their primary caregiver. Advika described "disappearing" into books and school work, sometimes forgetting that she had a body at all, spending hours after school working on programming, sometimes late into the night. As a function of class privilege, and also privilege related to birth-assigned sex, they were able to access many programming resources including computers and additional classes. She would sometimes sell older computers, or her programming skills, and sometimes used this money to buy girl's clothing and gendered toys. However, since they sometimes used this money to buy additional boy's clothing, and games associated with boys, they weren't sure if this was a function of gender dysphoria. She also enjoyed having a penis and felt perhaps this meant that she was not really trans.

In college, Advika joined the LGBT alliance, but continued to feel conflict regarding sexual attraction to people of many genders. Because they felt "womanly," they decided they must be gay and would frequently have risky and degrading sexual encounters with cisgender men, often athletes who were sexually closeted, and most of whom were white. With these partners, she described experiencing microaggressions and verbal abuse as a function of both white supremacy and cisheteronormativity. However, Advika avoided other BIPOC, and especially other immigrants from India, due to what they described as a lack of discretion around sexual identity in the community and also due to disdain and internalized anti-immigrant bias.

Advika largely attributed their trauma symptoms to an index trauma of having been mugged and verbally and physically assaulted while returning to their dorm room after a frat party. Her assailant used racist and anti-immigrant slurs during the attack; Advika also felt there was a gendered element to this based on her perceived femininity. However, over time it became clear that, while this experience had been painful and disruptive in Advika's life, emotional maltreatment and microaggressions were more central to their symptom profile.

When I first met Advika, I was aware of our similarities, particularly around gender and sexual identity in that we both identified under the broad umbrella of queer. I was also aware of our significant differences. We had differences in racial identity (Advika is BIPOC, I am white), citizenship status (Advika was navigating the immigration system of the United States and I am a citizen), age (Advika was almost 20 years younger than me, and attuned to youth culture and online culture in many ways I am not), and ability status (Advika was physically abled with a psychological disability, I am physically disabled and psychologically abled; neither of us was diagnosed with a developmental disability). We also had readily apparent differences in socioeconomic status, religious identity, size, and the languages we were raised in. All of these became apparent to me over the course of our intake session, but of course there was a great deal for me to learn about Advika that was only hinted at in the intake process. As a general rule, I don't ask much about trauma exposure in an intake, as safety has not yet been established, and establishing safety first is part of the clinical model I embrace. (I also have the luxury of not being in an environment that requires a comprehensive trauma history at intake. This works well for me, although would not work well for all providers.) So, while some of the details of Advika's trauma exposure emerged in our first meeting, the history reported here was gathered over many sessions, and sometimes Advika would surprise me with a new disclosure, or by returning to something we had talked about with new specificity of a new perspective. This is typical of how trauma work evolves for me.

Daniel

Daniel initially presented to my office with a very clear goal: he wanted a letter of support for top surgery. He did not believe ongoing psychotherapy could be useful to him, but he was prepared to tolerate it if required to meet his goal. This typified Daniel across the board—he was goal-driven and very contained. Thus, it took some time for me to recognize the degree of his anxiety.

In our first meeting, Daniel disclosed that he was "a man who happened to be of transgender experience." He had close-cropped hair and was dressed with military precision, and I was not surprised when he told me that he had recently retired from the US Navy after completing 20 years of service, dating back to junior ROTC in high school. In meeting him, I presumed that Daniel was African-American, although he quickly corrected me when I asked. "I'm Black," he asserted when I asked about his racial and ethnic identification.

Once Daniel had completed his contract with the Navy, some of his first actions after separation were to formally change his name and the gender marker on his identification, begin hormone treatment, and obtain an older set of men's dress whites (dress whites were recently made unisex). "I was so tired of people calling me ma'am," he told me, "I almost didn't make it to retirement." Daniel had known he was a man for years and had come to terms with living in an environment that was structurally hostile to his gender identity. He did not come out as transgender during the Obama-era lifting of the ban on trans military forces serving openly and described being very glad that he hadn't, as he retired under a more hostile administration and recognizes that he would have been targeted if he had come out when he was able. That said, he was clear that the years of living in a gender that was not his gender had taken a significant toll on him.

Daniel was the oldest of three brothers. He grew up in a Midwestern American home where fitness and athleticism were important values and described honing his skills as an athlete playing 2-on-2 versions of basketball, football, soccer, and baseball with his brothers and father. The family also enjoyed camping and hiking, and Daniel's father was explicit that these activities were preparation for military careers for the children. Daniel's father was also career Navy, as was one of his brothers (the rebel had joined the Air Force). The family also belonged to a Protestant church with a Black congregation, and church-related activities were the primary focus of Sundays in their home.

Daniel's mother died in a house fire when he was 2 years old. His father began a relationship with the woman who helped raise Daniel shortly thereafter. Daniel's stepmother had an infant from another relationship, and later she and Daniel's father had a child together. Daniel described a close and loving relationship with his stepmother, although they struggled in his adolescence as she wanted him to take an interest in women's clothing and in his hair, which he kept short. Daniel also described colorism directed at him in his home and community. He was (and remains) darker than his brothers, and his stepmother would sometimes express disappointment that "the only girl" in the family was dark. She occasionally suggested he use skin-bleaching cream and asserted that growing his hair long and using a chemical relaxer (or investing in wigs) would help him feel more attractive. Daniel encountered this style of conjoint colorism and gender policing at school and church as well as at home and grew up worrying that his choice of clothing, activities, and hairstyle might indicate that he was a lesbian, which he found very anxiety-provoking. It also felt confusing to him, as he knew he was attracted to men from an early age.

Daniel had been impacted by what he initially described as an ongoing sexual and romantic relationship with a significantly older cisgender man he met through JROTC activities while in the ninth grade. This relationship was something of an open secret in his community, and Daniel believes his parents had mixed feelings about it, but were ultimately also relieved that he was in a relationship with a man.

Ultimately, I gathered that the stressors that Daniel would identify as traumatic were losing his mother at an early age, anti-trans and anti-Black bias in the military, and several instances of military sexual assault, starting with the experiences described above. He was not sure if he thought of his adolescent experiences with the older man as assaultive, although definitely recognized that the differences in age, rank, and power lent themselves to coercion in that relationship. Much, much later in our work together, he disclosed that he believed he had been sexually abused by a male uncle in childhood, and that this may have left him particularly vulnerable to exploitive relationships later in life. Daniel also identified the strained relationship with his stepmother since coming out as a stressor, noting that she used the wrong pronouns and name for him about half the time, and described her grief at the loss of the girl she had imagined him to be. Daniel's father and brothers, however, got on board with his name and pronouns fairly rapidly, and he was out to his family for years before leaving the military and beginning medical transition.

Daniel was not sure that he wanted ongoing therapy, and I assured him that this was not a requirement for a letter of readiness for top surgery. Near the end of our assessment, I asked him if he used alcohol or other substances in a way that was concerning to him. He inhaled sharply and abruptly broke eye contact. "If I do, does that mean I don't get that letter?" he asked. "If you do, it might be a good thing to talk about," I replied,

> and you should certainly let your surgeon know. If you are struggling with alcohol use, the expectation is that your use is 'reasonably well-controlled,' but you should know that my willingness to write a letter of support for top surgery is not contingent on your sobriety.

I can't say he exactly unwound, as I never saw Daniel unwind, but he did soften somewhat. "My use is well-controlled," he said. "*Very* controlled."

"It seems like control is pretty important to you," I said (probably running my fingers through my unruly hair while sitting in an undisciplined fashion). "Do you think it might be helpful to talk more about that? You can come back if you'd like. But in any case I'll send a letter to your surgeon by the weekend," I added quickly. He decided, seemingly to his own surprise, that he would like to return the following week. I agreed to hold the time for him, not at all sure that I would see him again.

In my initial meeting with Daniel, I was aware of our similarities in age, socioeconomic status we were raised with, and that we were both AFAB and on the masculine spectrum. We were both American, although from very different parts of the country, and both communicate exclusively in English day-to-day. We also shared a similar dry sense of somewhat morbid humor, but I'm not sure I recognized that at first. Our immediately apparent differences were in racial identity, body morphology (Daniel was military muscular and I am not), positionality relative to the gender binary, sexual identity, religious background, and disability status.

Shai

Shai presented to my office explicitly wanting to work on symptoms related to trauma exposure, was not especially interested in talking about gender, and from our first interaction wanted to know my religious identity and my experience working with religious trauma. I was forthright in telling Shai that I had worked with TGD people from a variety of religious backgrounds, many of whom had experienced anti-trans bias in their home congregations, and that I myself am not religious. Shai also asked me if I was raised in a religious home, and specifically if I was raised Jewish. I disclosed that I was raised in an interfaith home with some Jewish members and some members of other faiths, and that I have never identified as Jewish. It was not until I got to that final disclosure that I observed Shai's body relax a little, although only a very small amount. They continued to retreat into my large office chair, as far away from me as it was possible to sit. Shai is living in a larger body, and their body is in a near-constant state of retraction and withdrawal. They often gave the impressions that they were further from me than it was physically possible to be, and I noted how frequently I felt as if I were shouting across a chasm trying to reach them.

Raised in in an Orthodox Jewish home on the east coast of the United States, Shai had experienced conversion therapy, in the guise of religious counseling, from their rabbi when their same-sex attraction became evident. Shai participated in this to the best of their ability from the age of seven, trusting and praying that the attraction would abate, and pushing themself to fantasize about "appropriate" partners as suggested by their rabbi. This attraction only grew stronger as adolescence unfolded, and Shai also noticed growing discomfort with the gender-segregated services offered in their shul. At age 14, they began to make shame-filled and clandestine trips to a nearby LGBT center, where they encountered a variety of different perspectives related to religious identity, sexual identity, and gender identity. Although terrified to be in this milieu, Shai quickly came to recognize that they desperately needed access to these different perspectives, and they began sometimes skipping scheduled extracurricular activities in order to spend more time at the center. During this process of exploration, Shai began to recognize that they are nonbinary, and primarily attracted to other nonbinary and gender diverse people. They were preparing to come out to their parents as they were coming to the realization that they could no longer attend conversion therapy nor could they continue to attend a shul that was segregated by gender. However, Shai was kicked out of their parents' home, at the age of 15, before they had the chance to disclose these personal revelations. An acquaintance saw them entering the LGBT center while holding hands with another nonbinary person and informed their parents, who reacted by angrily insisting that Shai leave immediately, asserting that they needed to protect Shai's younger siblings. Shai expressed frustration and grief about having been outed, not because they were unprepared for the aftermath, but because they were deprived of the opportunity to come out in their own time and their own way.

Upon being kicked out of their home, Shai spent several months as a homeless teen, usually sleeping on the couches of friends or sex partners from the LGBT center, but sometimes in parks or on rooftops. They described being mugged and "slapped around" while sleeping in a park and sexually assaulted when discovered on a rooftop, after which they became increasingly desperate for a steady place to live. Shai found their way into a shelter for LGBTQ teens and young adults and received help finding transitional housing. Having an address to use on employment applications made it possible for them to obtain a job in food service. With this identified source of income, they were able to become an emancipated minor at age 16. They augmented their verifiable income with income from work in the underground economy, generally camming (the performance of on-camera sex acts for money) or selling sex, although sometimes selling marijuana and cocaine to their co-workers. These years were very difficult for Shai, and they were at constant risk of additional trauma. They had past experiences with therapy, specifically group-based cognitive-behavioral therapy and dialectical behavioral therapy, while in the shelter system, but found it unhelpful at the time, in part because they were simply not in a safe environment. They were not at all convinced that therapy could be useful to them, but they were growing increasingly desperate. Their life had become more stable, in that they had housing, a job working as an overnight janitor for a company that provided cleaning services for offices, and regular clients for sex work. But with this stability had come an increase in symptoms and distress.

Shai identified as white, culturally Jewish, anti-religious, neurodivergent, fat, nonbinary, pansexual and aromantic, and as a sex worker. They were experiencing an array of symptoms related to traumatic stress, some of which they knew were trauma-related and some of which they did not. In my initial meeting with Shai, I was aware of our whiteness, and our similarities in embracing gender and sexual identities that do not center the binary. We also both had experiences with anti-fat bias. Additionally, I also left home very early, although under different circumstances, and could relate to a lot of what Shai had to say about self-reliance as well as their very factual assessment of risk and reward. For Shai, some of their factual assessment in this way was also a manifestation of their neurodivergence, and they were sometimes significantly more concrete than I am (and also much more rule-oriented). Developing a greater understanding of neurodivergence at the intersection of gender identity and traumatic stress exposure was helpful to me in my work with Shai.

IN SUM

I hope this chapter elucidates some of the many ways in which TGD people are at increased risk for exposure to trauma and stress. While I believe a solid grounding in exposure base rates, and comparisons to cisgender groups, can be useful, I also feel it is helpful to have a more clinically oriented lens for recognizing the various ways in which trauma-related sequelae can manifest. We will be following Advika, Daniel, and Shai through the rest of this manuscript as a way to represent the people behind the research numbers.

WORKS CITED

Ashley, F. (2022). *Banning Transgender Conversion Practices: A Legal and Policy Analysis.* UBC Press.

Austin, A., Herrick, H., & Proescholdbell, S. (2016). Adverse childhood experiences related to poor adult health among lesbian, gay, and bisexual individuals. *American Journal of Public Health, 106*(2), 314–320.

Barr, S. M., Snyder, K. E., Adelson, J. L., & Budge, S. L. (2021). Posttraumatic stress in the trans community: The roles of anti-transgender bias, non-affirmation, and internalized transphobia. *Psychology of Sexual Orientation and Gender Diversity.* Advance online publication.

Beckman, K., Shipherd, J., Simpson, T., & Lehavot, K. (2018). Military sexual assault in transgender veterans: Results from a nationwide survey. *Journal of Traumatic Stress, 31*(2), 181–190.

Blondeel, K., De Vasconcelos, S., García-Moreno, C., Stephenson, R., Temmerman, M., & Toskin, I. (2018). Violence motivated by perception of sexual orientation and gender identity: A systematic review. *Bulletin of the World Health Organization, 96*(1), 29.

Bond, M. A., Stone, A. L., Salcido Jr, R., & Schnarrs, P. W. (2021). How often were you traumatized? Reconceptualizing adverse childhood experiences for sexual and gender minorities. *Journal of Affective Disorders, 282,* 407–414.

Brömdal, A., Mullens, A. B., Phillips, T. M., & Gow, J. (2019). Experiences of transgender prisoners and their knowledge, attitudes, and practices regarding sexual behaviors and HIV/STIs: A systematic review. *International Journal of Transgenderism, 20*(1), 4–20.

Cannon, C. E. (2019). What services exist for LGBTQ perpetrators of intimate partner violence in batterer intervention programs across North America? A qualitative study. *Partner Abuse, 10*(2), 222–242.

Chang, T. K., & Chung, Y. B. (2015). Transgender microaggressions: Complexity of the heterogeneity of transgender identities. *Journal of LGBT Issues in Counseling, 9*(3), 217–234. doi:10.1080/15538605.2015.106

Exline, J. J., Przeworski, A., Peterson, E. K., Turnamian, M. R., Stauner, N., & Uzdavines, A. (2021). Religious and spiritual struggles among transgender and gender-nonconforming adults. *Psychology of Religion and Spirituality, 13*(3), 276–286. https://doi.org/10.1037/rel0000404

Galupo, M. P., Henise, S. B., & Davis, K. S. (2014). Transgender microaggressions in the context of friendship: Patterns of experience across friends' sexual orientation and gender identity. *Psychology of Sexual Orientation and Gender Diversity, 1*(4), 461.

Green, A. E., Price-Feeney, M., Dorison, S. H., & Pick, C. J. (2020). Self-reported conversion efforts and suicidality among US LGBTQ youths and young adults, 2018. *American Journal of Public Health, 110*(8), 1221–1227.

Griner, S. B., Vamos, C. A., Thompson, E. L., Logan, R., Vázquez-Otero, C., & Daley, E. M. (2020). The intersection of gender identity and violence: Victimization experienced by transgender college students. *Journal of Interpersonal Violence, 35*(23–24), 5704–5725.

Gyamerah, A. O., Baguso, G., Santiago-Rodriguez, E., Sa'id, A., Arayasirikul, S., Lin, J., … Wesson, P. (2021). Experiences and factors associated with transphobic hate crimes among transgender women in the San Francisco Bay Area: Comparisons across race. *BMC Public Health, 21*(1), 1–15.

Hilton, N. Z., Ham, E., & Green, M. M. (2019). Adverse childhood experiences and criminal propensity among intimate partner violence offenders. *Journal of Interpersonal Violence, 34*(19), 4137–4161.

James, S. E., Herman, J. L., Rankin, S., Keisling, M., Mottet, L., & Anafi, M. (2016). *The report of the 2015 U.S. transgender survey.* National Center for Transgender Equality.

Jenness, V., & Sexton, L. (2021). The centrality of relationships in context: A comparison of factors that predict the sexual and non-sexual victimization of transgender women in prisons for men. *Journal of Crime and Justice*, Advance online publication, 1–11.

Kroppman, C., Kim, S., Zaidi, A., Sharma, H., & Rice, T. R. (2021). Transgender and gender-nonconforming youth deserve further study in relation to adverse childhood experiences. *Journal of Gay & Lesbian Mental Health*, *25*(1), 2–4.

Miles-McLean, H. A., LaMotte, A. D., Williams, M. R., & Murphy, C. M. (2021). Trauma exposure and PTSD among women receiving treatment for intimate partner violence perpetration. *Journal of Interpersonal Violence*, *36*(13–14), NP6803–NP6826.

Mizock, L., & Lundquist, C. (2016). Missteps in psychotherapy with transgender clients: Promoting gender sensitivity in counseling and psychological practice. *Psychology of Sexual Orientation and Gender Diversity*, *3*(2), 148.

Morris, E. R., Lindley, L., & Galupo, M. P. (2020). "Better issues to focus on": Transgender microaggressions as ethical violations in therapy. *The Counseling Psychologist*, *48*(6), 883–915.

Murchison, G. R., Agénor, M., Reisner, S. L., & Watson, R. J. (2019). School restroom and locker room restrictions and sexual assault risk among transgender youth. *Pediatrics*, *143*(6), e20182902.

Nadal, K. L. (2018). Measuring LGBTQ microaggressions: The sexual orientation microaggressions scale (SOMS) and the gender identity microaggressions scale (GIMS). *Journal of Homosexuality*, 1404–1414.

Nadal, K. L., Skolnik, A., & Wong, Y. (2012). Interpersonal and systemic microaggressions toward transgender people: Implications for counseling. *Journal of LGBT Issues in Counseling*, *6*(1), 55–82.

Pulice-Farrow, L., Brown, T. D., & Galupo, M. P. (2017). Transgender microaggressions in the context of romantic relationships. *Psychology of Sexual Orientation and Gender Diversity*, *4*(3), 362.

Reisner, S. L., White Hughto, J. M., Gamarel, K. E., Keuroghlian, A. S., Mizock, L., & Pachankis, J. E. (2016). Discriminatory experiences associated with posttraumatic stress disorder symptoms among transgender adults. *Journal of Counseling Psychology*, *63*(5), 509–519.

Reuter, T. R., Newcomb, M. E., Whitton, S. W., & Mustanski, B. (2017). Intimate partner violence victimization in LGBT young adults: Demographic differences and associations with health behaviors. *Psychology of Violence*, *7*(1), 101.

Rodriguez, A., Agardh, A., & Asamoah, B. O. (2018). Self-reported discrimination in healthcare settings based on recognizability as transgender: A cross-sectional study among transgender US citizens. *Archives of Sexual Behavior*, *47*(4), 973–985.

Schnarrs, P. W., Stone, A. L., Salcido Jr, R., Baldwin, A., Georgiou, C., & Nemeroff, C. B. (2019). Differences in adverse childhood experiences (ACEs) and quality of physical and mental health between transgender and cisgender sexual minorities. *Journal of Psychiatric Research*, *119*, 1–6. https://doi.org/10.1037/cou0000143

Semiatin, J. N., Torres, S., LaMotte, A. D., Portnoy, G. A., & Murphy, C. M. (2017). Trauma exposure, PTSD symptoms, and presenting clinical problems among male perpetrators of intimate partner violence. *Psychology of Violence*, *7*(1), 91.

Shipherd, J. C., Maguen, S., Skidmore, W. C., & Abramovitz, S. M. (2011). Potentially traumatic events in a transgender sample: Frequency and associated symptoms. *Traumatology*, *17*(2), 56–67.

Smith, C. P., & Freyd, J. J. (2014). Institutional betrayal. *American Psychologist*, *69*(6), 575.

Stotzer, R. L. (2009). Violence against transgender people: A review of United States data. *Aggression and Violent Behavior*, *14*(3), 170–179.

Subirana-Malaret, M., Gahagan, J., & Parker, R. (2019). Intersectionality and sex and gender-based analyses as promising approaches in addressing intimate partner violence treatment programs among LGBT couples: A scoping review. *Cogent Social Sciences*, *5*(1), 1644982.

Thoma, B. C., Rezeppa, T. L., Choukas-Bradley, S., Salk, R. H., & Marshal, M. P. (2021). Disparities in childhood abuse between transgender and cisgender adolescents. *Pediatrics*, *148*(2), e2020016907.

Tobin, V., & Delaney, K. R. (2019). Child abuse victimization among transgender and gender nonconforming people: A systematic review. *Perspectives in Psychiatric Care*, *55*(4), 576–583.

Turban, J. L., Beckwith, N., Reisner, S. L., & Keuroghlian, A. S. (2020). Association between recalled exposure to gender identity conversion efforts and psychological distress and suicide attempts among transgender adults. *JAMA Psychiatry*, *77*(1), 68–76.

Wolfe, H. L., Boyer, T. L., Rodriguez, K. L., Klima, G. J., Shipherd, J. C., Kauth, M. R., & Blosnich, J. R. (2021). Exploring research engagement and priorities of transgender and gender diverse veterans. *Military Medicine*, Nov:usab460.

CHAPTER 5

PHYSIOLOGICAL FEATURES OF TRAUMA

Much of the contemporary physiological study of traumatic stress is in dialogue with Bessel van der Kolk's work, and particularly the book *The Body Keeps the Score: Brain, Mind and Body in the Healing of Trauma* (2014). An ever-expanding range of research literature indicates physiological differences between groups of people who have been exposed to traumatic stressors and those who have not, and people who meet diagnostic criteria for PTSD, and those who do not. There is evidence to suggest central and peripheral nervous system differences based on history of exposure to trauma and stress. There is also evidence to suggest physiological differences in trauma-exposed individuals with PTSD versus trauma-exposed individuals without PTSD. That is to say, populations that have not been exposed to traumatic stress have some population-level distinctions from people who have been exposed to traumatic stress, and among people who have been exposed to Criterion A stressors, there are population-level differences between those who develop PTSD and those who do not. While the focus in this manuscript is on the central nervous system and peripheral nervous system, as those are the systems with which I am most familiar, these differences are noted at every level of abstraction (e.g., differences can be seen from the genetic level to organism-wide) and in every major system of the body. These differences are also evident in physiological systems across time, including intergenerationally.

This chapter just scratches the surface of the body of literature related to physiological differences associated with trauma exposure. Several manuscripts synthesize this research, and many, many more could be written without capturing all of the pertinent information. The initial focus here will be on providing an overview of some of the ways in which psychophysiological data can be mis- and over-interpreted, including cautions to keep in mind when reading the research literature. We'll then move into discussing some of the unifying theories that seem to me to be most pertinent to the treatment of symptoms related to trauma and stress. As we go, we'll touch briefly on the physiological data that supports these theories. This is a bit different than many physiological overviews, which frequently start by covering the parts of the central and peripheral nervous systems. This can be useful grounding. However, as the focus of this manuscript is on clinical utility, I want to center the unifying theories rather than the approaches to measurement. I think it would be very interesting to provide a lot of information about electroencephalography (EEG), for instance, and through this ultimately arrive at a theory of information processing in PTSD. But I feel it may have clinical utility to talk about a theory of information processing in PTSD and then go on to discuss some of the EEG literature that supports theories of differential information processing in PTSD.

Since you may already be thinking, "Wow, this is a very subjective process," I'll start by acknowledging that this is a very subjective process. I want to be forthright about that, in part because it is my belief that all research is innately subjective. We develop hypotheses based on our preexisting ideas and questions, which are rooted in our experiences. Our experiences are an interaction of what we bring to the world around us and what the world around us brings back to us. Subjectivity, I would argue, is a feature of scientific research, not a bug. Our subjectivity is part of what drives research forward. Presenting research as

DOI: 10.4324/9781003140740-6

dispassionate or objective or separate from these personal processes is not actually objective, but rather comes from a place of disavowed subjectivity and unacknowledged privilege.

For the sake of increased transparency, then, I should acknowledge the places I am aware of having biases and preexisting ideas about psychophysiology and neurobiology. First, I love it. Second, I recognize that, like all research methodologies, it has limitations. My overarching difficulty with psychophysiology, and, indeed, with psychology in general is this: it's extractive and rooted in systems of domination. Labs and other medicalized settings (including psychotherapy offices, as we'll discuss later) are inherently white supremacist and cisheteronormative. By and large, they are not designed for BIPOC people, queer people, poor people, disabled people, or fat people. Even when BIPOC or queer or poor or disabled or fat people participate in research, the *systems* supporting the research are not designed for inclusion. Most, in fact, were actively designed for exclusion. In these circumstances, the research participants are generally being studied—usually by white, straight, cis, affluent, abled, thin people—to better understand how the participants' bodies, minds, and communities differ from the scientist's body, mind, and community, which the scientist has unwittingly internalized as "the norm." Once these data are collected, they are generally considered the intellectual property of the scientist. Once these data are decontextualized, aggregated, and analyzed, they will then typically be written about in a very specific format that is not intelligible to people who haven't had access to a particular kind of training, and the manuscripts submitted for publication in journals whose articles are behind paywalls. The process as it currently exists does not promote parity or collaboration between researchers and participants.

Nor does the process as it currently exists encourage people who are underrepresented in the sciences to feel comfortable imagining ourselves as researchers, thereby encouraging us to self-select out of these fields before getting started in them. Those of us who are underrepresented in the sciences and nonetheless *do* imagine ourselves as researchers often find our careers derailed due to the unexamined biases of senior scientists (see Kersey & Voight, 2020, for a grounded theory study on TGD graduate students in STEM; see Eaton et al., 2020, for research at the intersection of race and [cis]gender). I can say this based partially on my own experiences with a number of senior scientists, who very obviously enacted their biases with me over the course of my graduate training. This had an impact on my career trajectory, and on my sense of myself as a scientist.

As we go further into the sausage-making factory of psychophysiological research, I believe there are also some specific data analysis issues to consider, perhaps especially as relates to people who have experienced trauma and stress. First, almost all information derived from research articles utilizes means-based analysis in some way (for a theoretical overview of the limitations of means-based research in psychology, see Speelman & McGann, 2013). Although I believe that means-based analysis can be extremely useful for understanding physiological processes, there are a couple of caveats that are especially helpful to remember when we are considering the physiological reactivity of people who have been exposed to heightened stress or trauma. The first consideration is that physiological difference as a function of trauma exposure may fall into two distinct camps, and these two camps are associated with opposite patterns of psychophysiological response. For instance, if we were to take a group of people who had been exposed to trauma or stress, and we played some trauma-related audio recordings for them, some of them would likely experience an increase in their heart rates (and perhaps other elements of a fight/flight response), and others would likely experience a decrease in their heart rates (and perhaps other elements of a freeze/fawn response). People who have not been exposed to trauma might not show a change in heart rate at all while listening to these recordings. If we use the mean heart rate change from the trauma-exposed group and compare it with the mean heart rate change in the non-exposed group, it might look as if neither group experienced a change in heart rate because the increases in some trauma-exposed people are balanced out by the decreases in other trauma-exposed people. Thus, the trauma-exposed group *in aggregate* would look like the non-exposed group, but the trauma-exposed group would have a bimodal distribution of heart rate changes while the non-exposed group would more reflect the normal curve. (For a meta-analysis that speaks to this problem, see Pole, 2007.)

Another data-related consideration to keep in mind when interpreting the results of physiological studies is the way in which complex and evolving change is collapsed over time. When we compare means in most physiological studies, including neurobiological studies that utilize functional magnetic resonance imaging (fMRI), our means are extracted from data that are obtained across multiple time points. We might get a "baseline" mean of activation in a specific brain region across ten minutes in which we ask the participant to do nothing much, then have the research participant participate in a task of interest for ten minutes. (This is usually repeated a few times so as to have "baseline" blocks and "task" blocks.) We then collapse the resulting data (and it is a huge amount of data) down to a baseline mean for a region or network of interest and a task mean for a region or network of interest for each participant. We then collapse that data again for a baseline mean and a task mean for the control group, and a baseline mean and a task mean for the group of interest. A lot of the nuance of reactivity is lost in this process. This is important partly because the body is constantly engaged in the process of remaining in a narrow homeostatic band through a complex dance of *homeodynamics*. (I was first introduced to the term homeodynamics via the work of Lloyd et al., 2001, and it has greatly shaped my thinking about physiology and also clinical processes.) When you are startled, for instance, and your heart rate increases, this is partly because the processes that normally keep it lower are less active, and partly because the processes that speed it up are more active. Very quickly, however, the processes that bring your heart rate *down* become more active. This happens in order to keep your heart rate within the fairly narrow band of heart rate that sustains human life. These processes aren't restricted to your heart and vasculature. Other systems are recruited into the effort of managing your heart rate, and those systems, too, have fine-tuned calibrations that impact one another. But although we sometimes experience the moment of being startled as the start of this process, this complex interplay of systems doesn't have a start point or an end point. There is never a moment of homeostasis. There is only ongoing change across multiple systems with each system impacting, and being impacted by, the function of every other system, all of the time. This makes it difficult to know what we're really talking about when we talk about a psychophysiological "baseline." It also makes it difficult to know what, from a psychophysiological perspective, is a reaction to the psychological stimulus, and what is a homeodynamic response to the reaction.

Two final considerations for interpreting body-based research, particularly psychologically oriented brain imaging research, come to mind. The first is that it is very tempting for those of us producing and consuming brain-based research to fall into the trap of thinking that something is real because we can "see it in the brain" or "it changes the brain." The purpose of the brain is to change its pattern of activation in relationship to internal and external stimuli. In other words, everything changes the brain. This is amazing and wonderful. It indicates that brains are almost endlessly flexible and adaptable. But it does also mean that "we can see it *in the brain*" does not carry the weight of incontrovertible evidence for a theoretical construct. The whole point of brains is to change. Brains change much more readily than do minds.

Speaking of minds, the second brain-based consideration I want to offer is that brain activity does not map onto psychological phenomena in the way that we sometimes suggest. The brain, as far as I understand it, is fundamentally a bunch of on/off switches. As you may remember from a biological psychology class, if a neuron is sufficiently chemically activated, it fires. This firing is a brief electrical blip of "on." Many connected neurons turning "on" in different patterns are associated with different physiological and psychological phenomena. (If you have seen the child's toy Lite Brite, I'd say that the brain is basically a multidimensional Lite Brite.) So, when we say, for instance, that fMRI reveals that the insula is associated with disgust, what we really mean is that, when a person engages with stimuli that they report (or we believe) elicits the feeling of disgust, we observe increased blood flow in the insula that suggests a bunch of switches in the insula turned on. As researchers and consumers of research, we try to make sense of what we observe by constructing a narrative about which parts of the brain, or which networks of the brain, "do" various psychological phenomena. But the way the brain works (on/off switches) is different than the way psychological phenomena work (gradients, nuance, and complexity). So, while our narratives may be useful, and may even have some descriptive accuracy, it's probably counterproductive to get too confident in them. For an emotion-specific discussion that is adjacent to this, Lisa Feldman Barrett's *How Emotions Are Made: The Secret Life of the Brain* is an interesting read.

THEORIES OF HOW OUR BODIES RESPOND TO STRESS AND TRAUMA

There are a few things we know—or think we know—about how human bodies respond when in the midst of a traumatic or stressful experience. In this context, I am using traumatic or stressful to mean anything that overwhelms the individual's capacity for non-emergency coping, so the stressors will look different from person to person. However, our bodies tend to respond in fairly uniform ways when we are overwhelmed, and there are some ideas about what these uniform responses mean. One that I find clinically useful is that of the defense cascade. The defense cascade suggests that humans, like non-human animals, traverse a predictable cycle of arousal and activation when faced with threat (for a psychophysiologically intensive overview, see Lang et al., 1997; for a psychophysiological overview that provides clinical examples, see Kozlowska et al., 2015). When we believe threat may be imminent, we become watchful (as evidenced by activation in the visual cortex), hypervigilant (characterized by increased activation of the sympathetic nervous system or SNS), and enter a state of attentive immobility or active "freeze" (Kozlowska refers to this particular freeze state as fight-or-flight deferred). Active freeze includes an increase in respiration and heart rate, and an increase in muscle tone as the body begins to prepare for action, although some researchers note a decrease in heart rate at this juncture that is termed "fear bradycardia" (see Hamm, 2020). Once the threat becomes clear and imminent, we may have a fight-or-flight response that is generally characterized by additional sympathetic activation. During fight-or-flight, our digestion slows, blood is redirected toward larger striated muscles in our bodies, and epinephrine and norepinephrine are secreted into our bloodstream (which both heightens the general SNS effects and also seems to impact memory; see Elzinga & Bremner, 2002). There is evidence to suggest that the prefrontal cortex, which is associated with abstract cognition, becomes less active, while the limbic system (particularly the amygdala and the hippocampus), which is associated with strong emotion and survival-based responding, becomes more active (for an overview of the role of the prefrontal cortex and limbic system in PTSD, see Kredlow et al., 2022). However, depending on the individual, the nature of the threat, and possibly the proximity of the threat, we may instead have a different kind of freeze response, one of tonic (rather than attentive) immobility. This type of immobility is characterized by parasympathetic nervous system (PNS) dominance, including a lack of heart rate increase or a decrease in heart rate. In this form of immobility, there is downregulation of amygdala-based brain activity (i.e., the individual may experience less fear), and an increase in endogenous opioids (i.e., the individual will experience less pain). The individual may experience dissociative effects and be incapable of independent movement (for an overview of the relationship between increased prefrontal activity, or emotion overmodulation, and dissociation, see Lanius et al., 2010). There are elaborations on the model of the defense cascade, including differentiating between several different types of immobility (Volchan et al., 2017, e.g., differentiate between immobility under attack, with reduced heart rate, and tonic immobility, with increased heart rate). Some clinicians also incorporate what is called the "fawn" response, or avoiding attack through obsequiousness and accommodation at the expense of self. The fawn response has less research data to support it, but I find the construct very interesting, especially when we think about it in the context of intraspecies interactions (e.g., human-to-human). Fight-flight-freeze has largely been studied in prey responding to predator, but what happens when the big scary thing stalking toward you is also your source of comfort, or a family member you'll also have to see tomorrow? Perhaps, although not necessarily, a fawn response.

Clinically, I find an understanding of the defense cascade helpful in a variety of ways. First, it is useful for psychoeducation. It can help people understand why they are constantly on-edge and hyper-alert, attending to the possibility of threat at the expense of engaging in other activity. Understanding tonic immobility can also help people understand why they didn't fight back when abused or attacked. Knowing that endogenous opioids are released during tonic immobility has also helped me understand why so many people who have experienced significant trauma and stress insist that it "wasn't that bad." In the moment, their body's opioid system protected them from knowing how bad it was. Finally, while the defense cascade is something we generally think of as taking place in the moment of exposure to trauma or stress, it sets the stage for understanding longstanding differences in psychophysiology that might persist in survivors long after a traumatic incident itself is over.

While I would imagine that what we know about the defense cascade could be extended to TGD people, I can't say for sure, as these studies have not been completed. There is some data to indicate differences in psychophysiological responding to threat cues based on assigned sex at birth; specifically that cisgender men show a psychophysiological response more associated with attentive freezing while cisgender women show a psychophysiological response more associated with fight-or-flight (for a study of white cisgender students at University of Salzburg, see Wilhelm et al., 2017). However, these studies do not generally control for trauma exposure, so it is difficult to know if this is an assigned-at-birth sex difference, a sociocultural difference, or a trauma exposure difference. I could imagine it would also be interesting to focus on the fawn response specifically in TGD people, operating from the hypothesis that a fawn response could potentially look like performing in the gender role associated with their birth-assigned sex in order to evade harm or reduce tension in the home. However, these studies have yet to be conducted.

THEORIES OF HOW WE FUNCTION WHEN
IMPACTED BY TRAUMA AND STRESS

As mentioned above, the defense cascade is generally activated during moments of perceived threat, although of course some people are either threatened or perceive threat all of the time. When the defense cascade gets normalized into everyday life, to my mind the cycles of arousal most closely map on to a theory known as the window of tolerance (first described by Siegel, 1999; for a clinically focused overview, see Corrigan et al., 2011). The window of tolerance model suggests that there is a zone of optimal physiological arousal, in which a person is able to respond effectively to a variety of stimuli. An individual in the zone of optimal arousal (e.g., the window of tolerance) would be able to respond appropriately to a loud noise of unknown origin, for instance. When someone has experienced significant stress or trauma, their body will spend less time (or no time) in their personal window of tolerance. In this case, a loud noise might elicit a SNS-dominant reaction such as unchecked rage, or a flashback. Or it might elicit a PNS-dominant reaction such as numbness and dissociation (Siegel describes these as rigid versus chaotic responses and does not specifically relate them to traumatic experiences). Although many people tend to be more dominant in one response than another, homeodynamics make it physiologically difficult to be *entirely* sympathetic-dominant or parasympathetic-dominant. Instead, people who have experienced trauma and stress will often cycle through these physiological states, shifting between over-activated and under-activated and rarely in a "just right" state. Clinically, this theory can offer a useful metric in formulation—I will often consider whether I think someone is generally SNS-dominant, generally PNS-dominant, or wildly swinging between the two. This can guide the choice of interventions. Some people need interventions that are upregulating to their nervous systems in order to move into the window of tolerance, while some people need interventions that are downregulating to their nervous systems to move into the window of tolerance. And sometimes what worked yesterday is not going to work today, and we'll have to try some other things before we find an intervention that helps today.

Another way of understanding the neurobiology of chronic stress and trauma starting in childhood is through the neurosequential model of development (NM; see Perry, 2009, 2020). Both in utero and after birth, our brains and bodies develop in a predictable, sequential fashion. At birth, for instance, most of us have developed the neural networks necessary for breathing, but not for abstract moral reasoning. The regions of the brain that manage respiration, largely found in the brainstem, develop in utero, while the regions recruited for abstract reasoning (mainly cortical) develop over the course of many years after birth. NM focuses on the development of four major brain regions: the brainstem, the diencephalon, the limbic system, and the cortex. Development starts with the brainstem, which is the (evolutionarily) oldest and arguably least complex, and continues up the chain to the cortex. Each of these has a sensitive period from a developmental standpoint, and each has inputs that are needed in those sensitive periods in order for full maturation of the region. NM makes two separate but related points about this biological process. First, even if an individual gets the full range of necessary inputs at just the right developmental phase for limbic development, for instance, their brains will not be able to fully utilize these inputs if they did not get the appropriate inputs for brainstem development and diencephalon development during the sensitive periods related to the brainstem and diencephalon. It's like building an amazing second floor of a house on top of a limited foundation and wobbly first floor.

Second, an intervention that is targeted at the developmental level at which the individual is struggling is going to miss the mark. *The intervention must be targeted to the developmental level before the level of noticeable difficulty.* If someone is struggling to learn to read, for instance, although this may appear to be taking place at the cortical level, the intervention should initially target the limbic level. We can't make meaningful changes to the stability of the second floor if the first floor is still wobbly. Clinically, this model has guided my thinking regarding the necessity of a safety phase of trauma treatment. During the sensitive period of brainstem development, the primary tasks are related to physical survival such as getting food and staying thermoregulated. Because humans have a comparatively long and helpless period of infancy relative to many other animals, all of this happens in the context of a caregiving relationship. Adults who are struggling with accessing hunger cues, struggle to notice when they are hot or cold, or don't sleep until they are dropping from exhaustion, may have some brainstem-level developmental tasks to attend to in the context of the caregiving relationship of therapy. Checking in about the capacity of our clients to notice and attend to physical cues, then, is an important part of building safety.

Another theory that I find clinically useful is the theory of information processing in PTSD (for an overview see Blekic et al., 2021). This theory suggests that people who have been exposed to trauma and stress have less attention, relative to non-exposed control groups, to bring to bear on neutral or positive stimuli, and more attention to bring to aversive or traumatic stimuli. Two people may be in the same grocery store, for instance, and one of them may be able to readily focus on finding the food they want while the other is preoccupied by what they perceive as threatening body language in a nearby shopper. This is theorized to be part of the maintenance of symptoms in PTSD and may also leave people who have had trauma exposure in the past more susceptible to developing trauma-related symptoms if faced with a new stressor. This operates on the group level as well—white, affluent people might feel very comfortable in an environment, such as a private college, that was designed for white, affluent people, but these can be very dangerous environments for BIPOC people and poor people. Cisgender men might feel comfortable in a dark parking garage; cisgender women may be on-edge and tachycardic.

One piece of the physiological data that support the information-processing hypothesis of PTSD is that there are differences in the P300 brainwave of people with PTSD versus people without. The P300 wave is an event-related potential (ERP) that is measured via EEG. It typically appears at around 300 ms after the event of interest is presented. The latency (how long it takes to appear) is considered an indicator of information-processing speed, while the amplitude (the size of the wave) is considered an indicator of the attentional resources someone has available to bring to awareness of the event of interest. There is a lot of research regarding the P300 wave in PTSD, and a recent study of cisgender adults who had experienced maltreatment in childhood found a difference in the amplitude of the P300, in that the moderate-to-high abuse group had a smaller amplitude of P300 overall, and a higher amplitude of what is called Slow Wave to negative events and not positive or neutral events (Letkiewicz et al., 2020). I myself am thinking clinically about information processing in PTSD when reflecting on my self-management and presence in the psychotherapy space. A person who has experienced trauma and stress is going to notice any small cue that I might be angry or grappling with a negative judgment. There are processes happening within 300 ms of an encounter that will help them notice this, whether they're conscious of noticing it or not. Once these processes have come into play, their attentional resources will be consumed with monitoring for potential danger, and it will be difficult for us to do anything else. Additionally, it will probably be worse (e.g., the person will be more preoccupied) if I have an angry or negative reaction and try to hide it, as disavowed anger is often even more dangerous than acknowledged anger. Those of us who work with people who have experienced trauma and stress should be particularly mindful about how we come to treatment and be thoughtful about seeking support and consultation in difficult times or around difficult interactions. If specific strategies for physiological self-management when activated would be helpful for you, see Resmaa Menakem's *My Grandmother's Hands: Racialized Trauma and the Pathway to Mending Our Hearts and Bodies,* particularly if you are Black, white, or a police officer (2017).

The piece of information processing that is perhaps more directly related to our clients themselves can be found in literature related to the default mode network (DMN) in individuals who have experienced trauma and stress. The DMN consists of several highly connected brain structures (the ventromedial prefrontal cortex, the dorsal medial prefrontal cortex, and the posterior cingulate cortex) that are more active when an individual is passively lying in an fMRI scanner, and less active when the participant is engaged in a task of cognition or attention (for an overview, see Raichle, 2015). It is sometimes considered the network that is activated during spontaneous cognition (such as when we're daydreaming), although a more nuanced description may be that of the DMN as the nexus of self-centered predictions about the world (Raichle, 2010). Speculation about the DMN mediating self-referential processes (including memory, future projections about the self, and the state of the embodied self) coupled with differences in the DMN in people with PTSD has led to a theory of DMN contributions to the symptom profile of PTSD (Lanius et al., 2020). Specifically, this theory suggests that the DMN mediates the ways in which trauma and stress impact the sense of self in people who have had traumatic and stressful experiences. This is clinically relevant to understanding the disruptions of self that we may see when we work with individuals who have had traumatic or stressful experiences, including the sense of being separate from themselves, diffusion of self, and difficulty accessing body-based awareness. Although this has yet to be tested, I could imagine that the role of the DMN could be explored in TGD people, perhaps especially TGD people with lower or higher degrees of body satisfaction, or perhaps longitudinally in people whose body satisfaction changes over time.

Yet another theory related to the neurobiology of trauma and stress is that of the cerebellar cognitive affective syndrome (CCAS; see Schmahmann, 2010). The cerebellum is a portion of the brain that is active during physical tasks and especially physical tasks that include complex sequencing and oscillatory processes. In humans, it's the part of the brain that is active when you stand on one foot and remove your other shoe, for instance. We know that when we start to learn new physical tasks, we develop new neural connections in the cerebellum and its efferents, and we know that people with insult or injury of the cerebellum struggle with the smooth performance of physically coordinated tasks. CCAS suggests a role for the cerebellum in cognition and affect as well. In other words, oscillatory processes in how we think and feel might also be regulated by the cerebellum. A compromised cerebellum, then, might contribute to affective overreacting to stimuli (e.g., having a flashback when faced with a trigger) or affective underreacting to stimuli (e.g., shutting down and dissociating when faced with a trigger). I find this theory clinically useful in part because it is quite hopeful. The cerebellum is one of the more plastic regions of the brain. There may be interventions targeting cerebellar upregulation that could be rapidly effective for trauma survivors with affective dysregulation—specifically, patterned physical movement, which creates new cerebellar synaptic connections. In regard to TGD people, I'd be interested to know how learning new movement patterns, specifically those associated with gender expression, would impact cognition and affect, as mediated by cerebellar functioning.

Just to underscore, while I imagine that many of these research findings will generalize to TGD people, I cannot say for sure. There is some psychophysiological and neurobiological data of TGD people, but the majority of it seems to come in two different flavors: looking for a brain-based biomarker of TGD identity and/or gender incongruence, or pre-and-post HRT studies that explore whether TGD people are more like members of their assigned at birth sex or more like members of their gender. Neither of these is my area of interest or expertise, so I cannot adequately evaluate the methodology. However, for a networks-based perspective, I found Uribe et al. interesting (2020). For a volumetric overview, see Clemmens et al. (2021) or Baldinger-Melich et al. (2020). There are some TGD-specific trauma-related physiological concerns that I would put on the table as areas for future research, if I had a scanner of my own. One is related to pain sensitivity, and particularly pain sensitivity of genitals and chest/breasts. Another area would be regarding hypervigilance and orienting to gender cues in both out and closeted TGD people.

If you are a researcher who has not worked with TGD people before, and you are interested in expanding your research, I strongly advise you to work with TGD collaborators, hire TGD lab assistants and consultants, read best practices for research with TGD populations (e.g., Tebbe & Budge, 2016), and take an approach of deep humility.

PHYSIOLOGICAL IMPRESSIONS OF THE CASE STUDIES

From a physiological perspective, my best guess would be that Advika's presentation was generally hypoaroused, and this hypoarousal contributed to her dissociative presentation. What this looked like phenomenologically was that when they started to think and talk about things that were more difficult, they slowed way down. Her words would trail off and she would stare off into space, sometimes for minutes on end, and then come back to the conversation at a different point. It wasn't solely their speech that slowed—Advika's breathing would taper off, and their hands would fall to their lap or their sides. I could usually tell when she was coming back because her fingers would start to twitch as if she were typing, and she'd apologize and tell me she'd been distracted by thinking about a particularly difficult piece of programming. They also mentioned that this happened fairly frequently in day-to-day life, that they had sometimes missed stops on public transit or gotten lost driving to work because they were focused on programming. I asked if she had this experience during body-focused activities, such as while eating, exercising, or having sex. "Oh, I never do those things," they replied with a laugh.

From time to time, she would come to session sporting a bruise or scrape, usually with no idea how she came to be injured. They described how easy it was for them to misperceive their location in space, which I witnessed when they opened my office door into their own cheek one day. Her fingers would sometimes land on the injuries from these misadventures when she was spacing out, and she would press into those bruises and emit a thoughtful "hmm." Days of the week and time of day were difficult for them to keep track of, which they attributed to living with one foot in India and one in California. Some of this difficulty was managed through a rigid system of calendaring with several tiers of alarms and reminders, but Advika did acknowledge that sometimes she missed work meetings or found herself at the office on the weekend.

Advika had conceptualized their ongoing hypoarousal as an issue of focus and had been prescribed medication for ADHD. She found stimulant medication helpful for work performance and for managing her many obligations, but found that it exacerbated her sense of distance from her body. For a long time, this was one of the things they liked about using stimulant medication.

While Advika may have experienced chronic hypoarousal, Daniel was chronically physiologically hyperaroused, which I can state fairly definitively because he monitored his heart rate with a "smart" watch. He used this to track his workouts, and in session, we talked about whether it would be helpful for him to use it to track the duration and physiological intensity associated with flashbacks and panic attacks. (For people who like data and control, this can be a helpful strategy, although it is a double-edged sword for people whose desire for control extends to restricting food intake or over-exercise, so proceed with caution.) Daniel liked data and was accustomed to tracking his physiology from weight training and using run tracking apps, so the leap to using wearable tech in this way was not a big one for him. Moreover, he monitored his heart rate fairly regularly in any case, as he was worried about his cardiac health. Although he exercised frequently and was muscularly developed, his resting heart rate hovered around 90 beats per minute, and when we talked about difficult topics could spike to 120. Because of his long military career, Daniel had been thoroughly medically assessed for much of his life and had at one point had a cardiac workup with a Holter monitor. After this came back with no atypical results, he stopped talking about his concerns with his commanding officer, worried that he would be deemed psychologically unfit for duty.

Phenomenologically, he would regularly report racing heart, shallow breath, and a constriction in his chest and throat. He almost always felt too hot, but with chronically cold hands and feet, an indicator that his blood was moving away from his extremities and concentrating in his core. His experiences with heavy exercise also may have contributed to his ability to tolerate chronic hyperarousal, and he reported feeling calmest during times in which his heart rate was elevated for obvious reasons—when he was running or lifting weights. When we first started working together, he did not take training rest days and would lift weights despite sometimes significant strains and pains.

Perhaps related to his hyperarousal, he would sometimes talk about his stress-related experiences in a somewhat pressured fashion. This was notable, as pressured speech was not a common part of his presentation—in fact, he frequently came across as physiologically calmer than he was. From the outside, it would have been easy to interpret his somewhat rigid and formal way of moving through the world as hypoarousal or simply an artifact of his military training. Perhaps because of this, he had been diagnosed with persistent depressive disorder shortly after he separated from the Navy. Although he was prescribed an antidepressant, this prescription was never filled.

In my work with Shai, I came to understand that, for them, it was really the rate of change rather than any particular level of arousal that was the most destabilizing. Phenomenologically, Shai would sometimes present with rapid and pressured speech, the external appearance of a racing heart (e.g., flushed and sweaty), fast breathing, and rapid hand movements that I came to recognize as stimming associated with sensory overwhelm in autistic and neurodivergent people. (Once I was able to recognize stimming in Shai, I became much more attuned to it in both Shai and in other clients, and Shai and I were able to notice together that stimming indicated it was time to slow down a disclosure, and simply attend to their body.) At other times, they would present as flat, disoriented, and completely disconnected from what was happening around them, with very delayed reaction times. This presentation did not vary from session-to-session or month-to-month, but rather within the context of single sessions, and sometimes flipping back and forth several times within a session. I believe this presentation had contributed to a longstanding diagnosis of bipolar disorder, despite the fact that their cycles of up-and-down were far too rapid for bipolar disorder, and they had never experienced a manic episode. They had been prescribed a number of mood stabilizers and antipsychotic medications, which they took intermittently depending on their mood, finances, and degree of hostility to the medical establishment.

Although it is speculation, I believe that if we had the opportunity to monitor Shai's psychophysiology while in therapy, we would have seen an ongoing battle between their sympathetic and parasympathetic systems. Instead of their heart-rate rising and their respiratory sinus arrhythmia dropping in preparation for fight/flight, for instance, I think we might have potentially seen these indicators operating at cross-purposes, rising and falling together, perhaps, rather than one falling as the other rose. Instead of prefrontal shutdown and limbic activation, or prefrontal activation and limbic shutdown, we might have seen intense limbic activity and intense prefrontal activation at the same time, or reduced activity in both regions at the same time, and perhaps reduced cerebellar activity over all. What would have been missing, I imagine, is the smooth reciprocity of oppositional systems working in harmony to produce homeodynamics, and instead we would observe disjointed and incoherent physiological responding.

IN SUM

I hope that this offers a sense of the ways in which theories of psychophysiology and neurobiology can be helpful in formulating TGD clients who are living with sequelae of exposure to trauma and stress. In the next few chapters, we will continue to investigate how TGD people who have experienced trauma and stress might initially present in your clinic, before discussing a variety of treatment methods for addressing uncomfortable physiological and psychological states in this population.

WORKS CITED

Baldinger-Melich, P., Urquijo Castro, M. F., Seiger, R., Ruef, A., Dwyer, D. B., Kranz, G. S., … Koutsouleris, N. (2020). Sex matters: A multivariate pattern analysis of sex- and gender-related neuroanatomical differences in cis-and transgender individuals using structural magnetic resonance imaging. *Cerebral Cortex, 30*(3), 1345–1356.

Barrett, L. F. (2017). *How emotions are made: The secret life of the brain.* Houghton Mifflin Harcourt.

Blekic, W., Rossignol, M., Wauthia, E., & Felmingham, K. L. (2021). Influence of acute stress on attentional bias toward threat: How a previous trauma exposure disrupts threat apprehension. *International Journal of Psychophysiology, 170*, 20–29.

Clemens, B., Votinov, M., Puiu, A. A., Schüppen, A., Hüpen, P., Neulen, J., … Habel, U. (2021). Replication of previous findings? Comparing gray matter volumes in transgender individuals with gender incongruence and cisgender individuals. *Journal of Clinical Medicine, 10*(7), 1454.

Corrigan, F. M., Fisher, J. J., & Nutt, D. J. (2011). Autonomic dysregulation and the window of tolerance model of the effects of complex emotional trauma. *Journal of Psychopharmacology, 25*(1), 17–25.

Eaton, A. A., Saunders, J. F., Jacobson, R. K., & West, K. (2020). How gender and race stereotypes impact the advancement of scholars in STEM: Professors' biased evaluations of physics and biology post-doctoral candidates. *Sex Roles, 82*(3), 127–141.

Elzinga, B. M., & Bremner, J. D. (2002). Are the neural substrates of memory the final common pathway in posttraumatic stress disorder (PTSD)? *Journal of Affective Disorders*, *70*(1), 1–17.

Hamm, A. O. (2020). Fear, anxiety, and their disorders from the perspective of psychophysiology. *Psychophysiology*, *57*(2), e13474.

Kersey, E., & Voigt, M. (2020). Finding community and overcoming barriers: Experiences of queer and transgender postsecondary students in mathematics and other STEM fields. *Mathematics Education Research Journal*, Online First, 1–24.

Kozlowska, K., Walker, P., McLean, L., & Carrive, P. (2015). Fear and the defense cascade: Clinical implications and management. *Harvard Review of Psychiatry*, *23*(4), 263–287. doi: 10.1097/HRP.0000000000000065. PMID: 26062169; PMCID: PMC4495877.

Kredlow, A. M., Fenster, R. J., Laurent, E. S., Ressler, K. J., & Phelps, E. A. (2022). Prefrontal cortex, amygdala, and threat processing: Implications for PTSD. *Neuropsychopharmacology*, *47*(1), 247–259.

Lang, P. J., Bradley, M. M., & Cuthbert, B. N. (1997). Motivated attention: Affect, activation, and action. In P. J. Lang, R. F. Simons, & M. Balaban (Eds.), *Attention and orienting: Sensory and motivational processes* (pp. 97–135). Lawrence Erlbaum Associates.

Lanius, R. A., Terpou, B. A., & McKinnon, M. C. (2020). The sense of self in the aftermath of trauma: Lessons from the default mode network in posttraumatic stress disorder. *European Journal of Psychotraumatology*, *11*(1), 1807703.

Lanius, R. A., Vermetten, E., Loewenstein, R. J., Brand, B., Schmahl, C., Bremner, J. D., & Spiegel, D. (2010). Emotion modulation in PTSD: Clinical and neurobiological evidence for a dissociative subtype. *American Journal of Psychiatry*, *167*(6), 640–647.

Letkiewicz, A. M., Silton, R. L., Mimnaugh, K. J., Miller, G. A., Heller, W., Fisher, J., & Sass, S. M. (2020). Childhood abuse history and attention bias in adults. *Psychophysiology*, *57*(10), e13627.

Lloyd, D., Aon, M. A., & Cortassa, S. (2001). Why homeodynamics, not homeostasis? *The Scientific World Journal*, *1*, 133–145.

Menakem, R. (2017). *My grandmother's hands: Racialized trauma and the pathway to mending our hearts and bodies*. Central Recovery Press.

Perry, B. D. (2009). Examining child maltreatment through a neurodevelopmental lens: Clinical applications of the neurosequential model of therapeutics. *Journal of Loss and Trauma*, *14*(4), 240–255.

Perry, B. D. (2020). The neurosequential model. In M. H. Teicher, O. Munkbaatar, A. N. Schore, K. Gatwiri, B. D. Perry, G. Kickett, ... & M. C. A. Malchiodi (Eds.), *The handbook of therapeutic care for children: Evidence-informed approaches to working with traumatized children and adolescents in foster, kinship, and adoptive care* (pp. 137–155). Jessica Kingsley Publishers.

Pole, N. (2007). The psychophysiology of posttraumatic stress disorder: A meta-analysis. *Psychological Bulletin*, *133*(5), 725.

Raichle, M. E. (2010). Two views of brain function. *Trends in Cognitive Sciences*, *14*(4), 180–190.

Raichle, M. E. (2015). The brain's default mode network. *Annual Review of Neuroscience*, *38*, 433–447.

Schmahmann, J. D. (2010). The role of the cerebellum in cognition and emotion: Personal reflections since 1982 on the dysmetria of thought hypothesis, and its historical evolution from theory to therapy. *Neuropsychology Review*, *20*(3), 236–260.

Siegel, D. J. (1999). *The developing mind: How relationships and the brain interact to shape who we are*. Guilford Publications.

Speelman, C., & McGann, M. (2013). How mean is the mean? *Frontiers in Psychology*, *4*, 451.

Tebbe, E. A., & Budge, S. L. (2016). Research with trans communities: Applying a process-oriented approach to methodological considerations and research recommendations. *The Counseling Psychologist*, *44*(7), 996–1024.

Uribe, C., Junque, C., Gómez-Gil, E., Abos, A., Mueller, S. C., & Guillamon, A. (2020). Brain network interactions in transgender individuals with gender incongruence. *Neuroimage*, *211*, 116613.

van der Kolk, B. A. (2014). *The body keeps the score: Brain, mind and body in the healing of trauma.* Viking Press.

Volchan, E., Rocha-Rego, V., Bastos, A. F., Oliveira, J., Franklin, C., Gleiser, S., … & Figueira, I. (2017). Immobility reactions under threat: A contribution to human defensive cascade and PTSD. *Neuroscience & Biobehavioral Reviews*, *76*, 29–38.

Wilhelm, F. H., Rattel, J. A., Wegerer, M., Liedlgruber, M., Schweighofer, S., Kreibig, S. D., … Blechert, J. (2017). Attend or defend? Sex differences in behavioral, autonomic, and respiratory response patterns to emotion–eliciting films. *Biological Psychology*, *130*, 30–40.

CHAPTER 6

PSYCHOLOGICAL FEATURES OF TRAUMA

In the previous chapter, we talked about the difference in physiological processes in people with trauma exposure and without, and in people with PTSD and without. And while I do think that understanding physiological processes is useful for understanding the sequelae of trauma exposure, in practice I recognize that most mental health providers are going to be more focused on the *psychological* manifestations of these reactions. Thus, in this chapter we'll begin by discussing trauma-related sequelae that are a combination of physiological and psychological processes, such as differences in sleep, food intake, and the processing of pleasure and pain. These are sometimes the core criteria of diagnoses (e.g., sleep disruptions as criteria for sleep disorders) and sometimes considered symptoms associated with diagnoses (e.g., hypersomnolence in depression). Then we'll turn toward clusters of sequelae that are described by psychological diagnoses, with a focus on those that are frequently associated with trauma exposure—notably, substance use disorders; depressive, anxious, and bipolar disorders; dissociative disorders; psychotic-spectrum disorders; and suicidality. From this listing, you may feel that I more or less believe that the entire DSM consists of sequelae of exposure to trauma and stress. That is, in fact, more-or-less my position. I think that most of what we call psychopathology makes perfect sense in the context of our experiences, and that the DSM is essentially a culturally specific guidebook to the difficulties trauma and stress can cause. Thus, I believe that trauma and stress should be assumed and potentially ruled-out by the process of diagnosis. This is the inverse of much diagnostic thinking, which assumes we should look to genetic risk or other forms of vulnerability other than trauma, and then potentially rule trauma back *into* the consideration of etiology.

I have come to conceptualize a traumagenic frame as consistent with the social model of disability psychology, which may or may not be part of your theoretical framework. Theories of disability psychology suggest that there are at least three models for constructing disability: the moral model, the medical model, and the social model (see Olkin, 2002). Diagnosing someone with a form of psychopathology means that we are, by definition, diagnosing them with a psychological disability, so I see disability psychology as broadly applicable in the realm of clinical work. People who view disability through the lens of the moral model typically formulate disability as punishment for a transgression or sometimes as a "cross to bear" that brings disabled people closer to saintliness. The medical model, which is currently the predominant model in the United States, considers disability as something the body (or mind) is doing wrong—that there is a malformation or defect that should be corrected through medical intervention. An expert, in the form of a doctor or therapist, takes responsibility for heroically fixing the disabled individual—that is, making them "normal" or as close to the normal ideal as possible. Our system of diagnosis is predicated on this model, and the model itself smacks of (white) saviorism and cisheteronormative ideology in addition to being literally defined by ableism. The social model of disability holds that disability is socially constructed. This locates disability-related stressors (lack of access, poverty, etc.) in the society rather than the individual, whereas in the medical model, the problem is firmly located in the disabled individual. If we were to have a DSM based on the social model of disability, perhaps our billing codes would consist of community-based problems like poverty, environmental inequality, or lack of access to food, and our work would look very

DOI: 10.4324/9781003140740-7

different. This might not be your understanding of the role of clinicians, however, and that's perfectly fine—clinicians with a wide range of perspectives can be helpful to a wide range of clients. But I do want to be transparent about my biases regarding the pluses and minuses of the choice we are making by focusing on the individual as the unit of change.

However, in our medicalized milieu, we *do* focus on the individual as the unit of change. Therefore, I'll briefly mention one other challenge of working within a diagnostic framework before diving right into the diagnostic framework. The process of diagnosis is the process of making a determination that X presentation is a normal and healthy adaptation to the environment, while Y presentation is pathological and the "symptoms" related to this presentation must be eradicated or controlled. But deciding what is normal and what is pathological is predicated on culture and experience. In the United States as it currently exists, normalcy is an extension of colonialist and white supremacist ideals, patriarchy, and cisheteronormativity. What we consider to be healthy functioning exists in a very narrow and particular window. Sure, individual experience plus individual risk and resilience factors equal affect, behavior, and cognition. But all of this is situated in larger systems of families, neighborhoods, regions, and nations, each with its own mores and prescriptions regarding "normalcy." We do, however, live in the society we live in, with the mores and prescriptions that it has. Clinicians who operate in the theoretical framework of feminist psychotherapy (see Brown, 2018 for an overview) would argue that, in this context, sometimes, the most helpful thing we can offer an individual is the capacity to make a *choice* about whether they want to acquiesce to, or stand in opposition to, social demands. Recognizing that the oppressive system exists, and choosing to function as the system requires while holding the recognition that the system, not the person, is the problem, can be agentive and empowering. While locating problems in the individual is, I believe, destructive, locating places of power and agency in the individual, while recognizing the *context* as an environment that limits power and agency, can be very useful. Feminist psychotherapy is not the only framework for locating places of agency in an oppressive social context, and we'll talk about feminist-of-color and disability justice frameworks more in Chapter 12.

COMBINED PROCESSES

As mentioned above, I tend to think there are several processes that split the space between the physical and the psychological. Those that stand out to me are the ability to sleep and feel rested, the ability to eat without discomfort and to notice hunger and satiety, and the ability to notice and interpret appetitive and aversive bodily sensations such as pleasure and pain.

Sleep

Sleep is a basic physiological need, and sleep deprivation is a form of torture. We also know that sleeplessness is bidirectionally associated with psychological processes such as anxiety, depression, and psychosis. A study of sleep health, as measured through sleep-diaries and nighttime actigraphy, found that exposure to childhood trauma predicted poorer sleep health in adulthood, even after controlling for current stress levels (Brindle et al., 2018). Poor sleep health may then mediate the relationship between childhood trauma and symptoms of depression (Hamilton et al., 2018) and suicidality (King et al., 2021) as well as the relationship between Criterion A stressor exposure and development and severity of symptoms of PTSD (Lies et al., 2021). A conceptual overview of the relationship between trauma-induced insomnia and PTSD symptoms argues that insomnia is not simply an associated feature of PTSD, but rather that fear of sleep arises in the context of posttraumatic fear of loss of control, and the occurrence of nighttime re-experiencing, often in the form of nightmares (Werner et al., 2021). A recent study examines the ways in which sleep is impacted by a variety of sociodemographic variables, including race, socioeconomic status, sex assigned at birth, and geographic region (Petrov et al., 2020).

There is also a literature related to sleep disturbance in TGD people. Part of this literature examines the role of hormones in sleep regulation, and particularly on the role of testosterone in obstructive sleep apnea (see, e.g., Gavidia et al., 2021; Robertson et al., 2019). Moreover, there are also studies identifying non-hormone related disruptions in the sleep health of TGD people. A qualitative study of sleep health and mental health in a TGD sample identified that mental health concerns (especially anxiety) were associated with poorer sleep health, and also that sleep was directly impacted by TGD identity, including identity-based worry, and the physical effects of gender-affirming practices such as chest binding (Harry-Hernandez et al., 2020). A cross-sectional study of college students in the United States and Canada found that TGD survey respondents were twice as likely as their cisgender counterparts to report poor sleep health, and almost four times as likely to report suicidality (poor sleep is a common predictor of suicidality; Hershner et al., 2021). Finally, an online survey of TGD individuals made an explicit link between sexual assault and sleeplessness in TGD people in the context of minority stress (Kolp et al., 2020).

Food intake

Eating less or more than our bodies need for physical sustenance can also be considered both physical and psychological. Food intake is a basic physiological need, and withholding food or force-feeding are forms of torture. We also know that food intake is bidirectionally associated with psychological processes like depression, anxiety, and disordered eating. People may eat more or less than their bodies need due to past deprivation or as a way to numb out and feel disconnected from their bodies. We sometimes also eat when we're not hungry in order to celebrate holidays or events, connect with family or culture, or simply because it feels good. And, although food consumption is different than weight or size, many, many people use food intake or restriction in attempts to exert control over their weight and size.

In talking about trauma-related difficulties surrounding food intake, we are generally talking about underconsumption, overconsumption, or difficulties with the process of digestion. It should be noted that any of these can occur in a body of any size; they might also all co-occur in a body of any size.

Food-related psychological diagnoses, including anorexia, bulimia, and binge eating disorder, were associated with adverse childhood experiences in a cisgender sample of 36,309 American adults, with sexual abuse and physical neglect predicting eating-related diagnoses in cisgender men, and sexual and emotional abuse predicting eating eating-related diagnoses in cisgender women (Afifi et al., 2017). Eating-related diagnoses have also been associated with PTSD and subthreshold PTSD in individuals exposed to Criterion A stressors (Braun et al., 2019). Digestive disorders such as inflammatory bowel disease (IBD), irritable bowel syndrome (IBS), and gastroesophageal reflux disease (GERD), as well as metabolic disorders such as diabetes, are also associated with exposure to trauma and stress, although the direction of causality is unclear. For instance, a recent study examined the relationship between

IBD and posttraumatic stress due to medical trauma incurred during treatment of the diagnosis (Taft et al., 2019). This study found that 32% of cisgender participants with IBD also met diagnostic criteria for clinically significant posttraumatic stress. Notably, about 12% of the original respondents were screened out of the study because they met criteria for PTSD prior to medical treatment for IBD. Another study found that childhood trauma predicted suicidality in cisgender adults with IBD (Tripp et al., 2021). Finally, a study of a Canadian sample of cisgender people with IBD found a relationship between physical and sexual abuse in childhood and the diagnosis of ulcerative colitis in adulthood (Fuller-Thompson et al., 2015).

There are a variety of gendered and racialized expectations about body shape and size that contribute to people attempting to manipulate their weight through their food intake (see Burke et al., 2020 for a conceptual overview and exploration of gaps in the literature). In TGD people, who experience disordered eating at two to four times the rate of cisgender people (Gordon et al., 2021), these gendered expectations around bodies may be more clearly articulated and consciously present. Women may overconsume in order to develop curves or underconsume to meet a white feminine ideal of thinness. Men may underconsume to avoid curves, and also in the hopes of lightening or eliminating menses (one study also suggests underconsumption in men may be related to gendered socialization and expectation related to birth-assigned sex; Diemer et al., 2018). People of all genders may underconsume due to pressures of white supremacy and the androgynous (thin) ideal, or as a form of exerting control, or a way to feel numb. People of all genders may overconsume as a way to feel numb or as part of a cycle of underconsuming and overconsuming.

In one TGD-focused sample, 15% of youth presenting to a gender clinic reporting elevated scores on an eating disorders screening questionnaire (Avila et al., 2019). This, the study suggests, is actually a vast underreporting of scope, as more than 60% of the youth surveyed described attempting to manipulate their weight through managing food consumption for the purposes of navigating gender expression, and this would not be captured by typical screeners of disordered eating. Eating concerns increase risk of suicidality in people of all genders, and in a sample of TGD youth, body dissatisfaction, and specifically, a desire to be a different weight, was predictive suicidality (Peterson et al., 2017).

Pleasure and pain processing

For people who have been exposed to trauma and stress, differentiating between pleasure and pain can be confusing. This is true to a certain extent for all humans, as painful touch and pleasurable touch varies largely in degree of intensity, and the line between what is painful and what is pleasurable is certainly not universal. (For an overview of the shared neurobiology, see Leknes & Tracey, 2008; humans have also explored this shared neurobiology in any number of hands-on ways throughout history.) A common co-occurrence of trauma and stress is nonsuicidal self-injury (NSSI) such as cutting. This is a symptom that many clinicians struggle to work with effectively, in part because many of us find it activating and have difficulty understanding the variety of purposes it might serve (for a thematic overview of this challenge with trainees, see De Stefano et al., 2012).

One study of cisgender individuals admitted to the hospital for NSSI found that ACEs were the only statistically significant predictor separating the group of first-time hospital admissions from individuals that had experienced multiple admissions for NSSI (Cleare et al., 2018). Exposure to four or more ACEs predicted multiple hospital admissions in this sample, and every additional ACE conferred an 11% additional risk. Another study examined the relationship between PTSD symptoms and NSSI in cisgender adolescent survivors of child-hood sexual abuse (Weierich & Nock, 2008). They found the predicted relationship between childhood sexual abuse and NSSI and found that the symptom clusters of re-experiencing and numbing independently mediated the relationship between childhood sexual abuse and NSSI in this sample.

The relationship between NSSI and exposure to trauma has been empirically validated in TGD samples as well. A sample of TGD youth in the United Kingdom reported, on the whole, much higher rates of NSSI than the adolescent population means, with childhood sexual abuse a significant predictor of NSSI (Rimes et al., 2019). Childhood sexual abuse was found to be higher in the AFAB individuals who participated in this study; this was reflected in the rates of NSSI of the young men (79%) and AFAB nonbinary (81%) participants. A cross-sectional study of American adolescents found that over 50% of the TGD youth sampled had engaged in NSSI in the past year, with physical and sexual abuse among the predictors that separated a group of NSSI-only respondents from a group of respondents who reported both NSSI and suicide attempts (Taliaferro et al., 2019). One study indicates that TGD people may also engage in NSSI as a function of gender dysphoria specifically (Jackman et al., 2018).

Perhaps in part because NSSI can feel especially frightening to clinicians working with people who have experienced trauma and stress, we can sometimes forget to assess for our clients' capacity to experience pleasure—even though negative alterations in mood or cog-nition is one of the symptom clusters of PTSD as it is currently defined. Psychological con-structs such as anhedonia (Olson et al., 2018) and hedonic interference (Frewen et al., 2012) have been associated with trauma-exposed populations—in lay terms these mean that it is hard to feel good or activate neural "reward pathways" when one has experienced trauma and stress. This can also mean a paradoxical *negative* feeling in reaction to things that would be pleasant for people who have not been exposed to trauma and stress. Sex is a very partic-ular form of pleasure, and one that many people with PTSD and trauma exposure struggle to enjoy. (For a review paper that suggests that arousal becomes interpreted as anxiety in PTSD, and indicates the shared biological systems, see Yehuda et al., 2015. This review is, alas, limited to cisgender men and cisgender women.)

There are several studies that note a relationship between the experience of anhedo-nia and other mental health challenges in TGD people. Depressive symptoms, including anhedonia, in the TGD youth group were predicted by gender incongruence in a study of American adolescents (Gower et al., 2018). Regarding sex and sexuality specifically, a study of western European TGD people that focused on sexual satisfaction regardless of whether or not the person had pursued bottom surgery found that the primary difficulties in this sam-ple were difficulties initiating and seeking sexual contact, and difficulties achieving orgasm (Kerckhof et al., 2019).

DSM DIAGNOSES THAT ARE FREQUENTLY COMORBID WITH TRAUMA EXPOSURE

When the trauma-related physiological responses described in Chapter 5, and the trauma-related combination physiological/psychological processes described above, come together, they contribute to the foundation of diagnosable psychological states. As we have discussed, sometimes this takes the form of PTSD or CPTSD, but there are a number of psychiat-ric diagnoses that are commonly diagnosed alongside PTSD or CPTSD, or sometimes in lieu of PTSD or CPTSD. I want to mention these because sometimes people present to our offices with many co-occurring difficulties, and sometimes a broad array of diagnoses as well. I generally find it most useful to conceptualize all of these as trauma-related sequelae and to share that impression with my clients. This not only can reduce some of the stigma and shame around co-occurring diagnoses, but it allows for the creation of testable hypotheses within the clinical space. By this, I mean that we can observe whether or not a diagnosis—substance use disorder, for instance—begins to feel less intractable when the trauma is treated. If so, then the substance use is probably at least partially related to symptom-management of difficulties arising from trauma exposure. That does not mean that treating trauma means the person's substance use (or depression, or bipolar disorder, etc.) just goes away. It does, however, provide a different frame for formulating the substance use, for understanding the purpose it might be serving, and for finding other strategies for serving that purpose.

Substance use disorders

Substance use disorders are strongly associated with trauma and stress. This is a bidirectional relationship: people who have been exposed to trauma and stress may use substances in order to manage their distress, while risky substance use (including participation in the informal economy through purchasing substances that have been illegalized) leaves an individual vulnerable to increased trauma exposure. This has a cultural component as well, and discussion of substance use in TGD communities should be nuanced with the realization that substance use has been normalized in LGBTQ+ communities for generations. This was in part due to social and legal pressure—it was in underground bars and speakeasies that queer people were able to find connection with one another. Non-gender-specific cultural components should also be considered when talking with clients about substance use. For instance, although BIPOC people and white people use cannabis at about the same rate, BIPOC people are much more likely to be incarcerated for the possession and use of cannabis, thereby compounding trauma and also economic inequality (it is almost impossible to obtain employment after a period of incarceration or even an arrest). Limiting the income of traumatized, substance-using individuals may then push people further into the informal economy and also disconnect them from more formal systems of care, making legal forms of medication inaccessible. This then increases both trauma exposure and substance use. Additionally, there are also culturally specific patterns of substance use related to the treatment of posttraumatic sequelae, which will be revisited in Chapter 10.

The relationship between substance use disorders and PTSD is well-documented in the literature, with lifetime rates of substance use disorders in people with PTSD ranging from 21% to 43% (Jacobsen et al. 2001). Among cisgender men with PTSD, alcohol use disorder is the most common co-occurring diagnosis, followed by mood disorders; this pattern is reversed in cisgender women. An epidemiological study of cisgender American adults utilized latent class analysis to develop profiles of respondents based on exposure to ACEs and on lifetime substance use (Cavanaugh et al., 2015). While being a member of the higher ACEs class was associated with membership in the high use substance use class, this was not universal—about 30% of the higher ACEs profile was in the lower substance use group. Substance use disorders have also been linked to PTSD (for neurobiologically focused review of potential shared risk factors, see María-Ríos & Morrow, 2020). Stress related to racism and white supremacy has also been identified as a risk factor in the development of substance use disorders (see, e.g., Skewes & Bloom, 2019).

In a community sample of TGD adults, researchers explored lifetime experiences of substance use treatment history and also lifetime substance use treatment history combined with current self-reported substance use (Keuroghlian et al., 2015). Researchers regressed these outcome measures on four risk factors, which consisted of demographic risk, gender-related risk, mental health risk, and socio-structural risk. They found that more than 10% of this sample reported substance use treatment at some point, and more than 7% reported substance use treatment at some point and also current substance use. Predictive mental health risk factors were lifetime exposure to intimate partner violence and lifetime PTSD, while the predictive socio-structural factor was housing instability. (There were also gender-related risk factors, including being on cross-sex hormones, which they associated with greater access to health care services including greater access to substance use treatment.)

Non-medical use of prescription drugs, as well as polysubstance abuse, were high in a community sample of TGD adults, with more than 26% endorsing lifetime use of prescription medicines in non-prescribed ways (Benotsch et al., 2013). This study reported that individuals misusing prescription medication were also more likely to endorse a lifetime history of polysubstance use. These outcomes were predicted by lower self-esteem, more experiences of discrimination, and more self-reported psychopathology in the form of depression and anxiety. This study did not assess for PTSD or trauma exposure (other than gender-based discrimination), however, so while it elucidates relationships between gender and substance use, it does not speak to the role of trauma. A review of the substance use literature that focuses on the TGD community notes that these studies tend to oversample multiply marginalized, multiply traumatized TGD individuals, and thus establishing a baseline of usage across the larger community is difficult (Connolly & Gilchrist, 2020). This critique could potentially be applied to the TGD literature more broadly.

Depressive, anxious, and bipolar disorders

The first iteration of the PTSD diagnosis categorized PTSD as an anxiety disorder, and PTSD continued to be classified as an anxiety disorder until the DSM-5, in which it was recategorized in the new diagnostic category of Trauma and Related Stressors. (With this change has come some controversy—for an argument for maintaining PTSD as an anxiety disorder, see Zoellner et al., 2011.) The relationship between trauma exposure and anxiety and mood disorders cannot be overstated, even as we move away from categorizing PTSD itself as an anxiety disorder. One study investigated comorbidity with both PTSD and CPTSD in a representative cisgender sample of over 1,000 trauma-exposed participants in the UK (Karatzias et al., 2019). Of respondents with PTSD, 48% reported major depressive disorder (MDD) and 30% reported generalized anxiety disorder (GAD). Among the participants who met criteria for CPTSD, 89% met criteria for MDD and 86% met criteria for GAD. Anxiety disorders and depressive disorders are not solely highly comorbid with PTSD and CPTSD, they also frequently co-occur with ACEs. A study based on international data from the World Health Organization found that, worldwide, ACEs were associated psychopathology in cisgender adulthood, with maladaptive family functioning (including mental illness of a parent, parental substance use, and family violence) the category of ACEs with the greatest predictive power (Kessler et al., 2010). This study found that, if ACEs were eradicated, there would be a 23% reduction in mood disorders and a 31% reduction in anxiety disorders worldwide. A review and meta-analysis of articles related to multiple ACEs and adverse health outcomes drew from 37 articles representing more than 250,000 cisgender research participants (Hughes et al., 2017). This study found that exposure to four or more

ACEs was associated with an increase in odds ratio of anxiety (3.7) and depression (4.4) as compared with no ACEs. Childhood trauma has also been associated with bipolar disorder (for a review consolidating understanding of the etiology of risk see Aas et al., 2016). Another study suggests that it is the mix of depressive, anxious, manic, and psychotic symptoms that typifies exposure to childhood maltreatment (van Nierop et al., 2015).

There is a significant body of literature indicating the TGD people endorse high rates of depression and anxiety, although as we have seen this is mitigated among individuals who are supported in their gender identity. A review of the TGD literature from 2015 to 2020 identified several studies that included evaluations for anxiety and depression, and reports the prevalence rates of depression ranging from 33% to 50% and anxiety from 27% to 63% (Paz-Otero et al., 2021). The authors note that this is 4–10 times higher than estimated prevalence in the general population. A study of TGD youth presenting for treatment at a gender clinic found that 33% of the sample met criteria for MDD, and 48% met criteria for GAD (Chodzen et al., 2019). This study notes that higher levels of internalized transphobia were associated with both diagnoses, and a lower level of appearance congruence with the individual's affirmed gender was associated with MDD. A study of TGD adults investigated the relationship between discrimination experiences (as separate from Criterion A stressors) and found a relationship between everyday discrimination, PTSD symptoms, and symptoms of depression (Reisner et al., 2016). This study also presents several sociodemographic factors, including visual nonconformity, birth-assigned sex, race, income, and housing instability. (For additional granularity related to sexual and gender identity, see Borgogna et al., 2019.) Additionally, more attributed reasons for discrimination were associated with both more experiences of discrimination and more symptoms of PTSD, speaking to the importance of evaluating for additive and exponential stress related to experiencing different forms of bias. Finally, a cross-sectional analysis of medical records found that adults who had been diagnosed with a gender-related disorder were significantly more likely to be diagnosed with a mood disorder or an anxiety disorder (among others) than a cisgender comparison group (Wanta et al., 2019).

Dissociative disorders

For many clients and clinicians, the word dissociation is associated with dissociative identity disorder (DID), which is the experience of having multiple self-states that may, or may not, act and feel very differently from one another, and that may, or may not, have awareness of one another. I have noticed a recent trend toward calling this form of dissociation "living as a system," or sometimes plurality, rather than DID, and this appears to be associated with destigmatizing multiple self-states, and also deprioritizing the goal of integration into a single self-state (instead focusing on maximizing the strengths of the system). While it has been suggested that systems are quite rare, I would currently want to withhold judgment on that, as it seems possible to me that the phenomenon seems very rare because we rarely look for it. That said, this form of dissociation is very much not my area of expertise (for a review of the literature and a discussion of the controversy surrounding the diagnosis, see Dorahy et al., 2014; for a case study involving a TGD system, see Mun et al., 2020). I am much more conversant with dissociation along the lines of depersonalization, derealization, or simple "zoning out," which is very common in trauma-exposed individuals. The DSM-5 nods to this reality by including a dissociative subtype of PTSD (D-PTSD), which includes persistent feelings of depersonalization and/or derealization in addition to meeting the other PTSD criteria (for an overview of the rationale for this change, see Lanius et al., 2012; for a critique of the distinction see Burton et al., 2018). As with the move away from categorizing PTSD as an anxiety disorder, this was a controversial change, and there are several different models for understanding the overlap between trauma exposure and symptoms of dissociation. A review of latent profile analysis and latent class analysis studies related to the overlap suggests that D-PTSD is discriminable from PTSD and consistently associated with childhood sexual abuse (Hansen et al., 2017).

There is limited research related to dissociative symptoms in TGD people, although what does exist suggests the rates of dissociation are quite high among individuals with gender dysphoria. One study, which examines the relationship between gender dysphoria, childhood trauma, depression, and suicidality, suggests that almost 30% of individuals with gender dysphoria also report some form of dissociation (Colizzi et al., 2015). Colizzi and colleagues also note that symptoms of dissociation are reduced after interventions that address gender dysphoria. One potential future area of research suggested by this study and by my own clinical experience would be to investigate dissociation as a buffer against feelings of gender dysphoria. In the exploration of trauma and dissociation, we sometimes talk about dissociation as an adaptive response to inescapable trauma and stress. I could imagine the same rationale might apply to the ongoing inescapable stress of a body that is chronically misperceived and misgendered. This hypothesis is somewhat supported by a cross-sectional study of trauma-exposed LGBTQ+ individuals that focused on symptoms of PTSD and dissociation as related to anti-LGBTQ+ discrimination (Keating & Muller, 2020). Among the TGD participants in this study, greater appearance congruence (e.g., feeling that one appears as one's gender) was associated with lower symptoms of both PTSD and dissociation.

Psychotic-spectrum disorders

Trauma and stress exposure are not always considered alongside psychosis, which is sometimes thought to be exclusively biologically driven rather than a biopsychosocial phenomenon. However, a review of the phenomenology and epidemiology of links between PTSD and psychotic-spectrum symptoms argues that there may be shared risk to both PTSD and psychosis and points out that the flashbacks and numbing associated with PTSD may be misidentified as the positive and negative symptoms of schizophrenia and vice versa (Seedat et al., 2003). In one study of cisgender people diagnosed with severe and persistent mental illness (SPMI), virtually all of the respondents reported exposure to at least one Criterion A stressor, and more 40% met criteria for PTSD (Mueser et al., 1998). These researchers noted that only 2% of the participants had PTSD documented as a diagnosis in their charts, however.

The possibility of a subtype of PTSD, PTSD with secondary psychotic features (PTSD-SP) has been considered, and a recent review article summarizes the genetic and biologic evidence for this differentiation (Compean & Hamner, 2019). This article also highlights risk factors—notably child abuse and war trauma—associated with psychosis. These authors also discuss cultural expectations as related to the diagnosis of psychotic-spectrum disorders. A recent longitudinal analysis of trauma exposure, PTSD, and psychosis across the lifespan in a cisgender sample of Swedish individuals notes high associations between exposure, PTSD, and psychosis (Allardyce et al., 2021). This study notes that PTSD is associated with 15 times the risk of psychosis but does not mediate the relationship between trauma exposure and psychosis. One of the interpretations of these results is that PTSD and psychosis may both be part of a spectrum of responses to exposure to trauma and stress exposure rather than distinct and separable entities.

A recent review of the literature regarding the prevalence of psychotic-spectrum symptoms in TGD people synthesizes prior research while also highlighting some of the biases that have been incorporated into existing studies (Barr et al., 2021). This review highlights the need for future research in an especially invisibilized domain of psychiatry.

Suicidality

While suicidality is not a diagnostic category in itself, consideration of suicidality factors into treatment of people of all genders who are experiencing psychological distress. Suicidality is high among trauma-exposed individuals, and perhaps uniquely predicted by PTSD (see Wilcox et al., 2009). A study of lifetime suicidal ideation and suicide attempts found that cisgender respondents reported a lifetime prevalence of suicidal ideation of 13% (Kessler et al., 1999). Respondents with PTSD were five times more likely to have experienced suicidal ideation than demographically matched individuals without PTSD (this was much lower than rates endorsed by individuals with mood disorders, and about comparable to the rates in individuals who endorsed drug addiction). In the meta-analysis, mentioned above, of symptoms related to ACEs, ACEs had the most predictive value for suicide attempts (Hughes).

Eighty-two percent of respondents to the 2015 United States Transgender Survey reported serious suicidal ideation at some point, with 40% having made a serious attempt (James et al., 2016). These rates were highest among Indigenous (50%), multiracial (47%), and Black (45%) respondents and also varied as a function of family support of gender identity. Among individuals who were out to the families they grew up with, 37% of those from supportive families and 54% of those with unsupportive families described lifetime suicide attempts. This, of course, does not capture the experience of TGD people who completed suicide, some of them before ever disclosing their gender identity.

A review of the literature regarding TGD suicidality found that reported ideation ranged from 37% to 83% and history of attempts ranged 10–44% (McNeill et al., 2017). Another review focused on demographic features associated with suicidality in TGD people found similar racial disparities to the 2015 USTS, with Indigenous/First Nations individuals reporting the most suicidal ideation and number of attempts and white individuals reporting the least (Adams & Vincent, 2019). This study also notes lower income and lower educational achievement among TGD people as compared to the national average. A longitudinal study of risk and resilience in TGD adults found that a decrease in victimization and discrimination over the course of the study predicted a decrease in the severity of suicidality from baseline to follow-up (Rabasco & Andover, 2021). Moreover, increased TGD community connectedness over the course of the study also predicted a decrease in severity. Finally, a study of a community sample of TGD adults found that history of sexual violence, history of homelessness, and feeling unsafe all predicted suicidality. Lack of safety emerged as the only statistically significant independent predictor when all three predictors were entered into the model (Drescher et al., 2021).

THE CASE HISTORIES

Having discussed diagnostic nosology in the abstract, let's briefly return to the cases for a diagnostic overview.

Advika met criteria for anorexia, depersonalization/derealization, and gender dysphoria. Although I originally believed she had difficulty with sleep, or perhaps would meet criteria for delayed sleep phase syndrome, she ultimately disclosed that she used (and sometimes misused) ADHD medication to control both her sleep cycle and her food intake. They had a longstanding diagnosis of ADHD, but it was difficult to know the extent to which their difficulty with focus and their use of ADHD medication were a function of depersonalization/derealization and gender dysphoria, and how much their lack of focus and use of ADHD medication were helpful for them in terms of managing depersonalization/derealization and gender dysphoria. Advika reported occasional passive suicidal ideation without intent or plan. In terms of differential diagnosis, I should note that Advika did not meet criteria for PTSD. While she did have an index trauma that met Criterion A, she did not experience physiological hyperarousal or intrusive memories related to the event.

Daniel struggled greatly with sleep, often passing the night in a recliner in front of his television in a state of semi-wakefulness. When he did sleep deeply, it was frequently for just a couple of hours and mediated by his alcohol consumption. Daniel would not have met criteria for an eating disorder, but his focus on food as fuel might have qualified him for a diagnosis of orthorexia (an obsession with "clean" eating). However, orthorexia is not currently a diagnosable concern. Daniel met criteria for PTSD, GAD, alcohol use disorder, and gender dysphoria. He always staunchly denied suicidal ideation, and I always took him at his word, although I leave open the possibility that he was worried that an admission of suicidality could potentially result in a loss of his right to legally own firearms in the state of Illinois, which was a risk he was not prepared to take. In terms of differential diagnosis, it would have been easy for me to overlook the PTSD because of the strength of his generalized anxiety. While he was forthcoming about his physiological hyperarousal and general worry, it took a long time for him to disclose trauma exposure. Although he experienced avoidance around sex and sexual activity (his primary trigger), he managed this with alcohol use and would probably not have described himself as sex avoidant when we met.

In the youth shelter system, Shai had received many diagnoses, including bipolar disorder, borderline personality disorder, schizoaffective disorder, polysubstance use disorder, binge eating disorder, GAD, and MDD with psychotic features. This is not uncommon for trauma-exposed individuals—people who have been diagnosed with PTSD are eight times more likely to have three or more comorbid diagnoses than people with other psychiatric diagnoses (Kessler et al., 1995). That said, the one diagnosis Shai did *not* receive in the youth shelter system was PTSD.

My initial assessment of Shai was CPTSD. Shai later disclosed that they identify as neurodivergent and together we talked about tools for diagnosing autism and whether or not a formal autism diagnosis would be useful for them. In our evaluation they also met criteria for binge eating disorder and dissociative disorder not otherwise specified. While NSSI, hedonic interference, and suicidality are not diagnostic categories, these were pieces of Shai's experience. Shai also experienced sleep disturbances and described polysubstance use as well as cannabis misuse. In terms of differential diagnosis, Shai did not meet criteria for gender dysphoria or gender incongruence, as they were simply a nonbinary person without the experience of incongruence between their gender and their body.

IN SUM

Diagnostic considerations are important to the field and play a (sometimes quite significant) role in how we approach treatment. PTSD and CPTSD are considered the two primary trauma-related diagnoses, and recognizing these in their various manifestations is a central part of trauma-informed treatment. Understanding the relationship between trauma and stress and other associated sequelae is also important. When we stratify based on exposure to trauma and stress, we begin to see that, for instance, different treatments for depression have different efficacy depending on whether or not the individual has a history of trauma exposure (e.g., Nemeroff et al., 2005).

You may be wondering why this chapter did not discuss the convergence between trauma and stress exposure and the diagnosis of borderline persinality disorder (BPD). While I debated including BPD in this chapter, it is ultimately a deeply interpersonal difficulty, and therefore I opted to leave a discussion of BPD as relates trauma for the next chapter, which focuses on interpersonal facets of trauma exposure.

WORKS CITED

Aas, M., Henry, C., Andreassen, O. A., Bellivier, F., Melle, I., & Etain, B. (2016). The role of childhood trauma in bipolar disorders. *International Journal of Bipolar Disorders, 4*(1), 1–10.

Adams, N. J., & Vincent, B. (2019). Suicidal thoughts and behaviors among transgender adults in relation to education, ethnicity, and income: a systematic review. *Transgender Health, 4*(1), 226–246.

Afifi, T. O., Sareen, J., Fortier, J., Taillieu, T., Turner, S., Cheung, K., & Henriksen, C. A. (2017). Child maltreatment and eating disorders among men and women in adulthood: Results from a nationally representative United States sample. *International Journal of Eating Disorders, 50*(11), 1281–1296.

Allardyce, J., Hollander, A. C., Rahman, S., Dalman, C., & Zammit, S. (2021). Association of trauma, post-traumatic stress disorder and non-affective psychosis across the life course: A nationwide prospective cohort study. *Psychological Medicine*, Open Access, 1–9.

American Psychiatric Association. (2013). *Diagnostic and statistical manual of mental disorders* (5th edition). American Psychiatric Association.

Avila, J. T., Golden, N. H., & Aye, T. (2019). Eating disorder screening in transgender youth. *Journal of Adolescent Health, 65*(6), 815–817.

Barr, S. M., Roberts, D., & Thakkar, K. N. (2021). Psychosis in transgender and gender non-conforming individuals: A review of the literature and a call for more research. *Psychiatry Research, 306*, 114272.

Benotsch, E. G., Zimmerman, R., Cathers, L., McNulty, S., Pierce, J., Heck, T., … Snipes, D. (2013). Non-medical use of prescription drugs, polysubstance use, and mental health in transgender adults. *Drug and Alcohol Dependence, 132*(1–2), 391–394.

Borgogna, N. C., McDermott, R. C., Aita, S. L., & Kridel, M. M. (2019). Anxiety and depression across gender and sexual minorities: Implications for transgender, gender non-conforming, pansexual, demisexual, asexual, queer, and questioning individuals. *Psychology of Sexual Orientation and Gender Diversity, 6*(1), 54.

Braun, J., El-Gabalawy, R., Sommer, J. L., Pietrzak, R. H., Mitchell, K., & Mota, N. (2019). Trauma exposure, DSM-5 posttraumatic stress, and binge eating symptoms: Results from a nationally representative sample. *The Journal of Clinical Psychiatry, 80*(6), 14848.

Brindle, R. C., Cribbet, M. R., Samuelsson, L. B., Gao, C., Frank, E., Krafty, R. T., … Hall, M. H. (2018). The relationship between childhood trauma and poor sleep health in adulthood. *Psychosomatic Medicine, 80*(2), 200.

Brown, L. S. (2018). *Feminist therapy*. American Psychological Association.

Burke, N. L., Schaefer, L. M., Hazzard, V. M., & Rodgers, R. F. (2020). Where identities converge: The importance of intersectionality in eating disorders research. *International Journal of Eating Disorders, 53*(10), 1605–1609.

Burton, M. S., Feeny, N. C., Connell, A. M., & Zoellner, L. A. (2018). Exploring evidence of a dissociative subtype in PTSD: Baseline symptom structure, etiology, and treatment efficacy for those who dissociate. *Journal of Consulting and Clinical Psychology*, *86*(5), 439.

Cavanaugh, C. E., Petras, H., & Martins, S. S. (2015). Gender-specific profiles of adverse childhood experiences, past year mental and substance use disorders, and their associations among a national sample of adults in the United States. *Social Psychiatry and Psychiatric Epidemiology*, *50*(8), 1257–1266.

Chodzen, G., Hidalgo, M. A., Chen, D., & Garofalo, R. (2019). Minority stress factors associated with depression and anxiety among transgender and gender-nonconforming youth. *Journal of Adolescent Health*, *64*(4), 467–471.

Cleare, S., Wetherall, K., Clark, A., Ryan, C., Kirtley, O. J., Smith, M., & O'Connor, R. C. (2018). Adverse childhood experiences and hospital-treated self-harm. *International Journal of Environmental Research and Public Health*, *15*(6), 1235.

Colizzi, M., Costa, R., & Todarello, O. (2015). Dissociative symptoms in individuals with gender dysphoria: Is the elevated prevalence real? *Psychiatry Research*, *226*(1), 173–180.

Compean, E., & Hamner, M. (2019). Posttraumatic stress disorder with secondary psychotic features (PTSD-SP): Diagnostic and treatment challenges. *Progress in Neuro-Psychopharmacology and Biological Psychiatry*, *88*, 265–275.

Connolly, D., & Gilchrist, G. (2020). Prevalence and correlates of substance use among transgender adults: A systematic review. *Addictive Behaviors*, 106544.

De Stefano, J., Atkins, S., Noble, R. N., & Heath, N. (2012). Am I competent enough to be doing this? A qualitative study of trainees' experiences working with clients who self-injure. *Counselling Psychology Quarterly*, *25*(3), 289–305.

Diemer, E. W., White Hughto, J. M., Gordon, A. R., Guss, C., Austin, S. B., & Reisner, S. L. (2018). Beyond the binary: Differences in eating disorder prevalence by gender identity in a transgender sample. *Transgender Health*, *3*(1), 17–23.

Dorahy, M. J., Brand, B. L., Şar, V., Krüger, C., Stavropoulos, P., Martínez-Taboas, A., … Middleton, W. (2014). Dissociative identity disorder: An empirical overview. *Australian & New Zealand Journal of Psychiatry*, *48*(5), 402–417.

Drescher, C. F., Griffin, J. A., Casanova, T., Kassing, F., Wood, E., Brands, S., & Stepleman, L. M. (2021). Associations of physical and sexual violence victimisation, homelessness, and perceptions of safety with suicidality in a community sample of transgender individuals. *Psychology & Sexuality*, *12*(1–2), 52–63.

Frewen, P. A., Dean, J. A., & Lanius, R. A. (2012). Assessment of anhedonia in psychological trauma: Development of the hedonic deficit and interference scale. *European Journal of Psychotraumatology*, *3*(1), 8585.

Fuller-Thomson, E., West, K. J., Sulman, J., & Baird, S. L. (2015). Childhood maltreatment is associated with ulcerative colitis but not Crohn's disease: Findings from a population-based study. *Inflammatory Bowel Diseases*, *21*(11), 2640–2648.

Gavidia, R., Dunietz, G. L., Matlen, L., Hershner, S., Stroumsa, D., Kaplish, N., & O'Brien, L. (2021). 417 Transgender hormone therapy and sleep-disordered breathing. *Sleep*, *44*(Supplement_2), A165-A165.

Gordon, A. R., Moore, L. B., & Guss, C. (2021). Eating disorders among transgender and gender non-binary people. In *Eating disorders in boys and men* (pp. 265–281). Springer.

Gower, A. L., Rider, G. N., Coleman, E., Brown, C., McMorris, B. J., & Eisenberg, M. E. (2018). Perceived gender presentation among transgender and gender diverse youth: Approaches to analysis and associations with bullying victimization and emotional distress. *LGBT Health*, *5*(5), 312–319.

Hamilton, J. L., Brindle, R. C., Alloy, L. B., & Liu, R. T. (2018). Childhood trauma and sleep among young adults with a history of depression: A daily diary study. *Frontiers in Psychiatry, 9*, 673.

Hansen, M., Ross, J., & Armour, C. (2017). Evidence of the dissociative PTSD subtype: A systematic literature review of latent class and profile analytic studies of PTSD. *Journal of Affective Disorders, 213*, 59–69.

Harry-Hernandez, S., Reisner, S. L., Schrimshaw, E. W., Radix, A., Mallick, R., Callander, D., ... Duncan, D. T. (2020). Gender dysphoria, mental health, and poor sleep health among transgender and gender nonbinary individuals: A qualitative study in New York City. *Transgender Health, 5*(1), 59–68.

Hershner, S., Jansen, E. C., Gavidia, R., Matlen, L., Hoban, M., & Dunietz, G. L. (2021). Associations between transgender identity, sleep, mental health and suicidality among a North American cohort of college students. *Nature and Science of Sleep, 13*, 383.

Hughes, K., Bellis, M. A., Hardcastle, K. A., Sethi, D., Butchart, A., Mikton, C., ... Dunne, M. P. (2017). The effect of multiple adverse childhood experiences on health: A systematic review and meta-analysis. *The Lancet Public Health, 2*(8), e356–e366.

Jackman, K. B., Dolezal, C., Levin, B., Honig, J. C., & Bockting, W. O. (2018). Stigma, gender dysphoria, and nonsuicidal self-injury in a community sample of transgender individuals. *Psychiatry Research, 269*, 602–609.

Jacobsen, L. K., Southwick, S. M., & Kosten, T. R. (2001). Substance use disorders in patients with posttraumatic stress disorder: A review of the literature. *American Journal of Psychiatry, 158*(8), 1184–1190.

James, S. E., Herman, J. L., Rankin, S., Keisling, M., Mottet, L., & Anafi, M. (2016). *The report of the 2015 U.S. transgender survey*. National Center for Transgender Equality.

Karatzias, T., Hyland, P., Bradley, A., Cloitre, M., Roberts, N. P., Bisson, J. I., & Shevlin, M. (2019). Risk factors and comorbidity of ICD-11 PTSD and complex PTSD: Findings from a trauma-exposed population based sample of adults in the United Kingdom. *Depression and Anxiety, 36*(9), 887–894.

Keating, L., & Muller, R. T. (2020). LGBTQ+ based discrimination is associated with PTSD symptoms, dissociation, emotion dysregulation, and attachment insecurity among LGBTQ+ adults who have experienced Trauma. *Journal of Trauma & Dissociation, 21*(1), 124–141.

Kerckhof, M. E., Kreukels, B. P., Nieder, T. O., Becker-Hébly, I., van de Grift, T. C., Staphorsius, A. S., ... Elaut, E. (2019). Prevalence of sexual dysfunctions in transgender persons: Results from the ENIGI follow-up study. *The Journal of Sexual Medicine, 16*(12), 2018–2029.

Kessler, R. C., Borges, G., & Walters, E. E. (1999). Prevalence of and risk factors for lifetime suicide attempts in the National Comorbidity Survey. *Archives of General Psychiatry, 56*(7), 617–626.

Kessler, R. C., McLaughlin, K. A., Green, J. G., Gruber, M. J., Sampson, N. A., Zaslavsky, A. M., ... Williams, D. R. (2010). Childhood adversities and adult psychopathology in the WHO World Mental Health Surveys. *The British Journal of Psychiatry, 197*(5), 378–385.

Kessler, R. C., Sonnega, A., Bromet, E., Hughes, M., & Nelson, C. B. (1995). Posttraumatic stress disorder in the National Comorbidity Survey. *Archives of General Psychiatry, 52*(12), 1048–1060.

Keuroghlian, A. S., Reisner, S. L., White, J. M., & Weiss, R. D. (2015). Substance use and treatment of substance use disorders in a community sample of transgender adults. *Drug and Alcohol Dependence, 152*, 139–146.

King, C. D., Joyce, V. W., Nash, C. C., Buonopane, R. J., Black, J. M., Zuromski, K. L., & Millner, A. J. (2021). Fear of sleep and sleep quality mediate the relationship between trauma exposure and suicide attempt in adolescents. *Journal of Psychiatric Research, 135,* 243–247.

Kolp, H., Wilder, S., Andersen, C., Johnson, E., Horvath, S., Gidycz, C. A., & Shorey, R. (2020). Gender minority stress, sleep disturbance, and sexual victimization in transgender and gender nonconforming adults. *Journal of Clinical Psychology, 76*(4), 688–698.

Lanius, R. A., Brand, B., Vermetten, E., Frewen, P. A., & Spiegel, D. (2012). The dissociative subtype of posttraumatic stress disorder: Rationale, clinical and neurobiological evidence, and implications. *Depression and Anxiety, 29*(8), 701–708.

Leknes, S., & Tracey, I. (2008). A common neurobiology for pain and pleasure. *Nature Reviews Neuroscience, 9*(4), 314–320.

Lies, J., Jobson, L., Mascaro, L., Whyman, T., & Drummond, S. P. (2021). Postmigration stress and sleep disturbances mediate the relationship between trauma exposure and posttraumatic stress symptoms among Syrian and Iraqi refugees. *Journal of Clinical Sleep Medicine, 17*(3), 479–489.

María-Ríos, C. E., & Morrow, J. D. (2020). Mechanisms of shared vulnerability to posttraumatic stress disorder and substance use disorders. *Frontiers in Behavioral Neuroscience, 14,* 6.

McNeil, J., Ellis, S. J., & Eccles, F. J. (2017). Suicide in trans populations: A systematic review of prevalence and correlates. *Psychology of Sexual Orientation and Gender Diversity, 4*(3), 341.

Mueser, K. T., Goodman, L. B., Trumbetta, S. L., Rosenberg, S. D., Osher, F. C., Vidaver, R., … Foy, D. W. (1998). Trauma and posttraumatic stress disorder in severe mental illness. *Journal of Consulting and Clinical Psychology, 66*(3), 493.

Mun, M., Gautam, M., Maan, R., & Krayem, B. (2020). An increased presence of male personalities in dissociative identity disorder after initiating testosterone therapy. *Case Reports in Psychiatry, 2020,* 8839984.

Nemeroff, C. B., Heim, C. M., Thase, M. E., Klein, D. N., Rush, A. J., Schatzberg, A. F., … Keller, M. B. (2005). Differential responses to psychotherapy versus pharmacotherapy in patients with chronic forms of major depression and childhood trauma. *Focus, 100*(1), 14293–14296.

Olkin, R. (2002). Could you hold the door for me? Including disability in diversity. *Cultural Diversity and Ethnic Minority Psychology, 8*(2), 130.

Olson, E. A., Kaiser, R. H., Pizzagalli, D. A., Rauch, S. L., & Rosso, I. M. (2018). Anhedonia in trauma-exposed individuals: Functional connectivity and decision-making correlates. *Biological Psychiatry: Cognitive Neuroscience and Neuroimaging, 3*(11), 959–967.

Paz-Otero, M., Becerra-Fernández, A., Pérez-López, G., & Ly-Pen, D. (2021). A 2020 review of mental health comorbidity in gender dysphoric and gender non-conforming people. *Journal of Psychiatric Treatment Research, 3*(1), 44–55.

Peterson, C. M., Matthews, A., Copps-Smith, E., & Conard, L. A. (2017). Suicidality, self-harm, and body dissatisfaction in transgender adolescents and emerging adults with gender dysphoria. *Suicide and Life-Threatening Behavior, 47*(4), 475–482.

Petrov, M. E., Long, D. L., Grandner, M. A., MacDonald, L. A., Cribbet, M. R., Robbins, R., … Howard, V. J. (2020). Racial differences in sleep duration intersect with sex, socioeconomic status, and US geographic region: The REGARDS study. *Sleep Health, 6*(4), 442–450.

Rabasco, A., & Andover, M. (2021). Suicidal ideation among transgender and gender diverse adults: A longitudinal study of risk and protective factors. *Journal of Affective Disorders, 278,* 136–143.

Reisner, S. L., White Hughto, J. M., Gamarel, K. E., Keuroghlian, A. S., Mizock, L., & Pachankis, J. E. (2016). Discriminatory experiences associated with posttraumatic stress disorder symptoms among transgender adults. *Journal of Counseling Psychology, 63*(5), 509.

Rimes, K. A., Goodship, N., Ussher, G., Baker, D., & West, E. (2019). Non-binary and binary transgender youth: Comparison of mental health, self-harm, suicidality, substance use and victimization experiences. *International Journal of Transgenderism, 20*(2–3), 230–240.

Robertson, B. D., Lerner, B. S., Collen, J. F., & Smith, P. R. (2019). The effects of transgender hormone therapy on sleep and breathing: A case series. *Journal of Clinical Sleep Medicine, 15*(10), 1529–1533.

Seedat, S., Stein, M. B., Oosthuizen, P. P., Emsley, R. A., & Stein, D. J. (2003). Linking posttraumatic stress disorder and psychosis: A look at epidemiology, phenomenology, and treatment. *The Journal of Nervous and Mental Disease, 191*(10), 675–681.

Skewes, M. C., & Blume, A. W. (2019). Understanding the link between racial trauma and substance use among American Indians. *American Psychologist, 74*(1), 88.

Taft, T. H., Bedell, A., Craven, M. R., Guadagnoli, L., Quinton, S., & Hanauer, S. B. (2019). Initial assessment of post-traumatic stress in a US cohort of inflammatory bowel disease patients. *Inflammatory Bowel Diseases, 25*(9), 1577–1585.

Taliaferro, L. A., McMorris, B. J., Rider, G. N., & Eisenberg, M. E. (2019). Risk and protective factors for self-harm in a population-based sample of transgender youth. *Archives of Suicide Research, 23*(2), 203–221.

Tripp, D. A., Jones, K., Mihajlovic, V., Westcott, S., & MacQueen, G. (2021). Childhood trauma, depression, resilience and suicide risk in individuals with inflammatory bowel disease. *Journal of Health Psychology, 27*(7), 1626–1634.

van Nierop, M., Viechtbauer, W., Gunther, N., Van Zelst, C., De Graaf, R., Ten Have, M., … Outcome of Psychosis (GROUP) investigators. (2015). Childhood trauma is associated with a specific admixture of affective, anxiety, and psychosis symptoms cutting across traditional diagnostic boundaries. *Psychological Medicine, 45*(6), 1277–1288.

Wanta, J. W., Niforatos, J. D., Durbak, E., Viguera, A., & Altinay, M. (2019). Mental health diagnoses among transgender patients in the clinical setting: An all-payer electronic health record study. *Transgender Health, 4*(1), 313–315.

Weierich, M. R., & Nock, M. K. (2008). Posttraumatic stress symptoms mediate the relation between childhood sexual abuse and nonsuicidal self-injury. *Journal of Consulting and Clinical Psychology, 76*(1), 39.

Werner, G. G., Riemann, D., & Ehring, T. (2021). Fear of sleep and trauma-induced insomnia: A review and conceptual model. *Sleep Medicine Reviews, 55*, 101383.

Wilcox, H. C., Storr, C. L., & Breslau, N. (2009). Posttraumatic stress disorder and suicide attempts in a community sample of urban American young adults. *Archives of General Psychiatry, 66*(3), 305–311.

Yehuda, R., Lehrner, A. M. Y., & Rosenbaum, T. Y. (2015). PTSD and sexual dysfunction in men and women. *The Journal of Sexual Medicine, 12*(5), 1107–1119.

Zoellner, L. A., Rothbaum, B. O., & Feeny, N. C. (2011). PTSD not an anxiety disorder? DSM committee proposal turns back the hands of time. *Depression and Anxiety, 28*(10), 853.

CHAPTER 7

INTERPERSONAL FEATURES OF TRAUMA

As we have seen, exposure to trauma and stress can contribute to differences in an individual's body and psyche. This has implications for how that person moves through the world, including their ability to engage socially, cognitively, and emotionally. It also impacts that person's ability to build positive relationships and community. Difficulty engaging with the larger interpersonal world limits the support the individual is able to obtain in the structural facets of life. Thus, individuals who have experienced trauma and stress may struggle to connect with family, friends, and intimate partners; they may also struggle to engage in higher-order systems such as systems of employment, education, healthcare, and social services. This is, like most things, multifaceted and multidirectional—the interpersonal struggles influence the support the individual is able to receive in these facets of life, which in turn helps reinforce the individual's ideas about trust, risk, affinity, and love. For instance, a person who is more likely to be bullied at school is less likely to trust teachers or administrators and also less likely to receive support from those teachers and administrators if they *do* ask for help. They then are less likely to ask for support in the future and more likely to drop out of school. This further limits their access to potentially positive interpersonal relationships as well as access to education and job training.

The last chapter began with a discussion of those places that are somewhat in-between physiological and psychological processes—sleeping, eating, and processing pleasure and pain. This chapter will begin with some places that I think straddle the line between psychological processes and interpersonal or environmental processes, beginning with the personality disorders, especially borderline personality disorder (BPD). We will then move to alexithymia and other difficulties with verbalization; differences related to social cognition, including evaluating risk and reward; and then to revictimization, polyvictimization, and perpetration of victimization. After considering these strands individually, I'll offer a conceptual overview of what these strands taken together might mean for those times in which TGD people who have been exposed to trauma and stress engage with hostile, cisheteronormative systems. Then we'll turn to the case histories for an overview of how all of this might look clinically and what it might mean for a therapeutic relationship.

PERSONALITY DISORDERS

Personality traits are thought to be patterns of perceiving and relating that are relatively fixed over time. Personality pathology is diagnosed when these patterns are so fixed and so poorly suited to the individual's environment that the disjuncture causes significant life friction, and most particularly difficulty in interpersonal relationships. Personality disorders are also highly stigmatized. A review of the literature found that stigma surrounding personality disorders, and especially BPD, is high among both clients and health care providers, and this can impact care (Ring & Lawn, 2019).

The primary model of personality-related diagnosis in DSM-5 is categorical, outlining diagnostic criteria for ten different personality disorders. BPD is the one that is most commonly associated with exposure to trauma and adversity, and a recent meta-analysis of

DOI: 10.4324/9781003140740-8

BPD and ACEs suggests that emotional maltreatment (both abuse and neglect) is the ACE category most predictive of this diagnosis (Porter et al., 2020). Antisocial personality disorder is also associated with ACE exposure, and particularly physical abuse (Gobin et al., 2015).

There is a dimensional alternative model of personality disorders under investigation in DSM-5, and this formulation closely mirrors that of the ICD-11 model, which consolidated all of the personality disorders into a single personality disorder diagnosis (see Pires et al., 2021, for an overview and comparison between the models). The DSM-5 dimensions are impairments in personality functioning (described as impairments in sense of self and impairments in interpersonal relatedness) and maladaptive personality traits (of which there are 25 traits in five domains; McCabe & Widiger, 2020). This is further specified as mild, moderate, or severe, and there is a borderline pattern qualifier. This model remains under review in the DSM-5, but I mention it because I find a dimensional approach to personality disorders more useful than the categorical approach, and because this alternative model captures the two dimensions relevant to this chapter: dimensions of the self and of the interpersonal. (For an overview of the ICD-11 criteria, with case-study applications, see Bach & First, 2018.)

The diagnosis of BPD has been so associated with trauma exposure that there is a body of literature arguing that CPTSD would be more parsimoniously diagnosed as co-occurring PTSD and BPD. This formulation has potential utility as a way to destigmatize some of the more interpersonally challenging elements of what is now considered to be BPD and also perhaps to share knowledge bases of trauma treatments that may be helpful for what is now called BPD as well as treatments for BPD that might benefit trauma survivors (Kulkarni, 2017). A recent latent class analysis suggests that there is separability between CPTSD and BPD in a highly traumatized cisgender sample, but that there was a great deal of overlap between the two, with impulsivity and temper outbursts offering the strongest differentiation (Jowett at al., 2020). I find myself in a place of being somewhat agnostic about how this question of diagnosis is resolved. My bias would be toward destigmatizing both diagnoses.

This is partially my bias because the stigma around BPD is especially pertinent to TGD people. Gender incongruence was, for many years, theorized to be a manifestation of the "unstable sense of self" of BPD, although BPD was sometimes instead described as a (near-inevitable) co-occurrence with gender incongruence rather than the diagnostic underpinning of gender incongruence (e.g., Meyer, 1982). Although this has shifted somewhat, clinicians should keep in mind that, while there are currently no mental health diagnoses that would definitively rule out gender-affirming medical interventions as an option, psychiatric symptoms must be "reasonably well-controlled" in order to move forward with gender-affirming medical interventions. Personality-related symptoms are considered, by many clinicians, to be especially difficult to manage or "control." It also seems possible to me that many clinicians may have unexplored biases that continue to conflate gender incongruence with personality-related symptoms. A recent study, for instance, utilized both the standard (categorical) and alternative (dimensional) DSM-5 models for understanding personality-related diagnoses in TGD people presenting to an Italian gender clinic (Anzani et al., 2020). The alternative model assessments were made based on a self-report questionnaire, while the standard assessments were based on clinician-administered clinical interviews. The diagnoses that came from the clinical interviews suggested significant personality pathology in this sample, while the self-assessments suggested low levels of personality-related symptoms. One interpretation of these data is that clinicians continue to view gender incongruence and/or TGD identities through the lens of personality pathology. For a review of ways in which gender minority stress may impact borderline symptoms, see Goldhammer et al. (2019).

ALEXITHYMIA AND VOICE

Alexithymia is described as difficulty labeling emotions and other internal states. People with alexithymia may find it difficult to describe what they are feeling or only be able to describe it in very basic terms (limited to "good" or "bad" for instance), even if they have an otherwise-expansive vocabulary. A meta-analysis of alexithymia in PTSD specifically found that alexithymia is common in PTSD, especially among cisgender men with combat-related PTSD (Frewen et al., 2008). Alexithymia has also been associated with ACEs. In a cisgender sample of Finns with Major Depressive Disorder, for instance, ACEs predicted difficulty in the "describing feelings to others" domain of alexithymia (Honkalampi et al., 2020).

Another trauma-related difference in vocalization or verbalization is in prosody. Prosody is the variation in our voices that allows us to add richness and layers to speech. A fluent speaker of a language or dialect can tell if the same sentence is sarcastic or sincere, spoken happily or in grief, because of the prosody. PTSD resulting from childhood trauma had the effect of reducing the ability to differentiate between joy, fear, and sadness (although not anger) from vocal prosody in a group traumatized cisgender women versus healthy controls, and the greater the trauma exposure the longer this differentiation took (Nazarov et al., 2015). Another study that focused on cisgender men who were veterans used naturalistic recording of these participants responding to questions from the Clinician Administered PTSD Scale and found that vocal elements such as more monotonous, flatter speech predicted PTSD (Marmar et al., 2019). Thus, it seems that exposure to trauma and stress impacts both the production of our own prosody and the recognition of prosodic elements in the speech of others.

I bring up the research related to verbal expression and trauma and stress in part because verbal expression has strongly gendered elements. Voice, and being gendered correctly in vocal communication, is very important to many TGD people. A voice that concords with the individual's gender predicted global assessment of quality of life in women (Hancock et al., 2011) and in men (Watt et al., 2018). A review of the elements of vocal presentation most relevant to TGD people found that prosody (defined in this study as intonation, tempo, and stress) was one of the three key factors for identifying gender through speech (Leung et al., 2018). Women and feminine-spectrum people with PTSD may find it more difficult to be heard as women as a function of social expectations about feminine prosody.

SOCIAL COGNITION AND ASSESSMENT OF RISK AND REWARD

The term social cognition has a variety of meanings and has been used to describe a number of different processes. It is sometimes used to describe empathy or theory of mind and sometimes to describe attachment-based relational processes. A review of the literature related to social cognition in PTSD, which focuses on the processing of social signals, found that groups with PTSD showed significant difficulty in tasks of social cognition relative to both healthy controls and trauma-exposed controls without PTSD (Stevens & Jovanovic, 2019). These researchers raise the question as to whether difficulty with social cognition is an outcome of PTSD, or a risk factor for developing PTSD after trauma exposure, and discuss the ways in which healthy social connection acts as a buffer against symptom maintenance in PTSD. Risk and reward systems, and systems of threat detection, are sometimes considered subsets of social cognition. People with PTSD experience less satisfaction from rewards and show a willingness to take greater risks than people without PTSD (for a review, see Seidemann et al., 2021).

There is little data about social cognition in TGD people, although there is a body of literature regarding how cisgender people think about and empathize with (or not) TGD people. One study measures implicit bias related to TGD people and finds implicit bias predicts levels of support for policy related to TGD people (Axt et al., 2021). Regarding risk and reward assessment in TGD people, much of the literature focuses on risk of HIV transmission (e.g., Poteat et al., 2015). A qualitative study of BIPOC women constructed a model through which the need for gender affirmation can contribute to risk behavior such as unprotected receptive anal sex and the use of hormones and body modification strategies accessible through informal networks (Sevelius, 2013). Although these confer greater risk of HIV transmission, this is weighed against the reward of gender affirmation and body satisfaction.

Although coping based on avoidance and approach is somewhat conceptually different than assessment of risk and reward, there is some similarity in the sense that a determination to approach or avoid can be understood as a function of assessment of risk and reward. A qualitative study of Black women identified themes of approach and avoidance among survivors of violence and found some parallels and some points of divergence from literature focused on cisgender women (Sherman et al., 2021). Approach themes in this study included some that are common in cisgender women such as help-seeking and acceptance. However, the researchers identified some themes that they described as unique to this particular sample. These included self-affirming behavior, in which the participants described seeking out ways to affirm their various identities (most particularly self-affirmation around gender expression) and self-protection such as code-switching and passing/blending.

REVICTIMIZATION, POLYVICTIMIZATION, AND PERPETRATION OF VICTIMIZATION

Revictimization is the experience of a similar trauma that is enacted by multiple perpetrators—for instance when an individual leaves a relationship with an abusive partner and then enters into a relationship with a different partner who is also abusive, or when an individual who was sexually abused as a child is sexually assaulted as an adult. PTSD symptoms are linked to revictimization, and this appears to be a bidirectional relationship, with revictimization experiences contributing to PTSD symptoms, and PTSD symptoms contributing to risk of revictimization (for an overview, see Jaffe et al., 2019). Revictimization has also been linked to ACEs. The odds of an adult who experienced four or more ACEs having experienced violence as an adult are more than seven times that of an adult who did not experience any ACEs (Hughes et al., 2017). This metric also points, less directly, to the phenomenon of polyvictimization. Polyvictimization is experiencing multiple types of victimization, whether by the same or other victimizers. Thus, an individual who endorses four or more ACEs has most likely *already* experienced polyvictimization, even if they are never revictimized in adulthood. (I say "most likely" because it is theoretically possible that an individual could endorse four ACEs related to family dysfunction and not have experienced direct victimization.) Polyvictimization is also associated with increased trauma- and stress-related distress (for an editorial and introduction to a special issue focused on polyvictimization, see Ford & Delker, 2018; and also Wolfe, 2018).

If further victimization is one element of initial victimization, perpetration of victimization is another element. According to the ACEs study cited above, experiencing four or more ACEs was associated with an eight times greater risk of perpetrating violence (Hughes). A meta-analysis examined patterns of victimization and perpetration among cisgender people in intimate partnerships, as related to patterns of mental health distress (Spencer et al., 2019). This meta-analysis indicated that PTSD and anxiety were more strongly correlated with victimization, while personality disorders were more strongly correlated with perpetration. Perpetration is seemingly at least partly also described by the phenomenon of identification with the aggressor, in which a victimized individual begins to take the position and perspective of the individual who is victimizing them (Lahav et al., 2022).

While rates of revictimization *per se* have not been extensively studied in TGD individuals, a recent meta-analysis of intimate partner violence (IPV) in relationships with one or more TGD individual found that, when compared with cisgender study participants, TGD study participants were 1.66 times more likely to have been in a relationship that included IPV, and this disparity was higher (2.89) among youth (Peitzmeier et al., 2020). Experiences of IPV were predicted by bullying, family assault and harassment, and other forms of victimization, indicating that the TGD people in this meta-analysis were at increased risk of experiencing both revictimization and polyvictimization, including multiple types of violence. This review also noted mixed findings related to whether or not TGD people perpetrated IPV more than cisgender people. One of the four studies mentioned in this meta-analysis that assessed for perpetration found that, among adults presenting to a community health clinic, the TGD sample endorsed higher rates of perpetration of IPV than the cisgender sample (Reisner et al., 2014). Regarding polyvictimization, a recent online study of adolescents of all genders found that 40% of the sample had experienced ten or more forms of victimization in the preceding year (Sterzing et al., 2017). Rates of polyvictimization were significantly higher among the TGD adolescents, however, with AMAB nonbinary (71.5%) and girls (63.4%) reporting the highest rates of polyvictimization. Boys (48.9%) and AFAB nonbinary (49.5%) also reported higher rates of polyvictimization when compared with cisgender peers. When focusing on adults, a secondary data analysis of the data from the 2015 USTS reports on five different violence types, and the likelihood of having experienced a greater number of violence types as a function of identity factors such as birth-assigned sex, gender, race, disability status, age, sexual identity, visual conformity with affirmed gender, and experience of being unhoused (Messinger et al., 2021).

TRAUMAGENIC ENVIRONMENTS

All of these factors taken together mean that TGD people are going to interact with the world in ways that cisgender people don't necessarily understand, and that people who have experienced trauma and stress will interact with the world in ways that the ways that people who have not had those experiences might not understand. Because of the ways in which revictimization and polyvictimization work (i.e., the ways in which trauma tends to "load" on people who have already experienced trauma—and especially people with multiple marginalized identities) TGD people who have experienced trauma and stress have probably experienced a *lot* of trauma and stress. You may encounter hostility, suspicion, rage, or what can seem like a very low frustration tolerance. On the other hand, you may notice a "too much, too soon" quality in your interactions with TGD people who have experienced trauma and stress, and notice that they are consistently putting their trust in untrustworthy people. You might observe difficulty navigating seemingly straightforward environments and sensitivity to perceived rejection.

We talked a great deal in Chapter 4 about the ways in which institutions fail TGD people, so I won't recapitulate that here. I do, however, want to comment on the ways in which talking about trauma "loading," as if it's happenstance or value-neutral, or something to do with the individual, is a formulation that lets us off the hook as a society. Animal models show us that the way to turn an ordinary adult rat with a litter of pups into a neglectful parent is to deprive that rat of resources (Ivy et al., 2008). Trauma loads because we, as a society, do not make resources available to people who need help, and then we pathologize, incarcerate, and scapegoat people when they have so much unmet need that it begins to inconvenience those of us who are hoarding the resources to begin with. When there is a lot of unmet need in a family or a community, the most vulnerable are going to suffer the most, and people who are suffering might not always act the way we like.

INTERPERSONAL CONSIDERATIONS IN THE CASE HISTORIES

In terms of interpersonal considerations, Advika initially came across to me as somewhat dramatic. She would often produce quite a lot of verbal content without really saying that much (producing what I sometimes think of as a wall of words). As described in Chapter 4, Advika had experienced polyvictimization and revictimization. They also ultimately described mocking, and sometimes verbally harassing, women and feminine-spectrum people while simultaneously suppressing their identification with the feminine spectrum.

Daniel seemed to me to be rather guarded and taciturn when we first started working together. This decreased somewhat over time, but his disclosures tended to either pour out of him in a way that left him feeling overwhelmed and shaken or come out after great deliberation and often after a great deal of testing my capacity to tolerate disclosures. Daniel had experienced chronic revictimization in the form of sexual violence.

Shai was, and is, angry. On an anger scale of 1–10, they are usually at an 8, and it takes very little to tip that into an 11. The task for me, especially in early sessions, was to simply withstand the blast. Shai had experienced polyvictimization and revictimization and continued to experience polyvictimization and revictimization for some time after initiating treatment. They also described perpetration of acts of psychological and physical violence against strangers, partners, and friends.

IN SUM

Over the past three chapters, we explored the physiological, psychological, and interpersonal effects that trauma can have. We have also been building diagnostic impressions of the people whose case histories are illustrating the various manifestations of these. The next two chapters will provide an overarching treatment framework, and then we will return to our case histories as we toward specific treatments and interventions in Chapters 10–12.

WORKS CITED

American Psychiatric Association. (2013). *Diagnostic and statistical manual of mental disorders* (5th edition). American Psychiatric Association.

Anzani, A., Panfilis, C., Scandurra, C., & Prunas, A. (2020). Personality disorders and personality profiles in a sample of transgender individuals requesting gender-affirming treatments. *International Journal of Environmental Research and Public Health, 17*(5), 1521. https://doi.org/10.3390/ijerph17051521

Axt, J. R., Conway, M. A., Westgate, E. C., & Buttrick, N. R. (2021). Implicit transgender attitudes independently predict beliefs about gender and transgender people. *Personality and Social Psychology Bulletin, 47*(2), 257–274.

Bach, B., & First, M. B. (2018). Application of the ICD-11 classification of personality disorders. *BMC Psychiatry, 18*(1), 1–14.

Ford, J. D., & Delker, B. C. (2018). Polyvictimization in childhood and its adverse impacts across the lifespan: Introduction to the special issue. *Journal of Trauma & Dissociation, 19*(3), 275–288. doi: 10.1080/15299732.2018.1440479

Frewen, P. A., Dozois, D. J., Neufeld, R. W., & Lanius, R. A. (2008). Meta-analysis of alexithymia in posttraumatic stress disorder. *Journal of Traumatic Stress, 21*(2), 243–246.

Gobin, R. L., Reddy, M. K., Zlotnick, C., & Johnson, J. E. (2015). Lifetime trauma victimization and PTSD in relation to psychopathy and antisocial personality disorder in a sample of incarcerated women and men. *International Journal of Prisoner Health, 11*(2), 64–74.

Goldhammer, H., Crall, C., & Keuroghlian, A. S. (2019). Distinguishing and addressing gender minority stress and borderline personality symptoms. *Harvard Review of Psychiatry, 27*(5), 317–325.

Hancock, A. B., Krissinger, J., & Owen, K. (2011). Voice perceptions and quality of life of transgender people. *Journal of Voice, 25*(5), 553–558.

Honkalampi, K., Flink, N., Lehto, S. M., Ruusunen, A., Koivumaa-Honkanen, H., Valkonen-Korhonen, M., & Viinamäki, H. (2020). Adverse childhood experiences and alexithymia in patients with major depressive disorder. *Nordic Journal of Psychiatry, 74*(1), 45–50.

Hughes, K., Bellis, M. A., Hardcastle, K. A., Sethi, D., Butchart, A., Mikton, C., … Dunne, M. P. (2017). The effect of multiple adverse childhood experiences on health: A systematic review and meta-analysis. *The Lancet Public Health, 2*(8), e356–e366.

Ivy, A. S., Brunson, K. L., Sandman, C., & Baram, T. Z. (2008). Dysfunctional nurturing behavior in rat dams with limited access to nesting material: A clinically relevant model for early-life stress. *Neuroscience, 154*(3), 1132–1142.

Jaffe, A. E., DiLillo, D., Gratz, K. L., & Messman-Moore, T. L. (2019). Risk for revictimization following interpersonal and noninterpersonal trauma: Clarifying the role of posttraumatic stress symptoms and trauma-related cognitions. *Journal of Traumatic Stress, 32*(1), 42–55.

Jowett, S., Karatzias, T., Shevlin, M., & Albert, I. (2020). Differentiating symptom profiles of ICD-11 PTSD, complex PTSD, and borderline personality disorder: A latent class analysis in a multiply traumatized sample. *Personality Disorders: Theory, Research, and Treatment, 11*(1), 36.

Kulkarni, J. (2017). Complex PTSD – A better description for borderline personality disorder?. *Australasian Psychiatry, 25*(4), 333–335.

Lahav, Y., Allende, S., Talmon, A., Ginzburg, K., & Spiegel, D. (2022). Identification with the aggressor and inward and outward aggression in abuse survivors. *Journal of interpersonal violence, 37*(5–6), 2705–2728.

Leung, Y., Oates, J., & Chan, S. P. (2018). Voice, articulation, and prosody contribute to listener perceptions of speaker gender: A systematic review and meta-analysis. *Journal of Speech, Language, and Hearing Research, 61*(2), 266–297.

Marmar, C. R., Brown, A. D., Qian, M., Laska, E., Siegel, C., Li, M., ... & Vergyri, D. (2019). Speech-based markers for posttraumatic stress disorder in US veterans. *Depression and Anxiety, 36*(7), 607–616.

McCabe, G. A., & Widiger, T. A. (2020). A comprehensive comparison of the ICD-11 and DSM–5 section III personality disorder models. *Psychological Assessment, 32*(1), 72.

Messinger, A. M., Guadalupe-Diaz, X. L., & Kurdyla, V. (2021). Transgender polyvictimization in the US Transgender Survey. *Journal of Interpersonal Violence*, 08862605211039250.

Meyer, J. K. (1982). The theory of gender identity disorders. *Journal of the American Psychoanalytic Association, 30*(2), 381–418.

Nazarov, A., Frewen, P., Oremus, C., Schellenberg, E. G., McKinnon, M. C., & Lanius, R. (2015). Comprehension of affective prosody in women with post-traumatic stress disorder related to childhood abuse. *Acta Psychiatrica Scandinavica, 131*(5), 342–349.

Peitzmeier, S. M., Malik, M., Kattari, S. K., Marrow, E., Stephenson, R., Agénor, M., & Reisner, S. L. (2020). Intimate partner violence in transgender populations: Systematic review and meta-analysis of prevalence and correlates. *American Journal of Public Health, 110*(9), e1–e14.

Pires, R., Henriques-Calado, J., Sousa Ferreira, A., Bach, B., Paulino, M., Gama Marques, J., ... Gonçalves, B. (2021). The utility of ICD-11 and DSM-5 traits for differentiating patients with personality disorders from other clinical groups. *Frontiers in Psychiatry, 12*, 343.

Porter, C., Palmier-Claus, J., Branitsky, A., Mansell, W., Warwick, H., & Varese, F. (2020). Childhood adversity and borderline personality disorder: A meta-analysis. *Acta Psychiatrica Scandinavica, 141*(1), 6–20.

Poteat, T., Wirtz, A. L., Radix, A., Borquez, A., Silva-Santisteban, A., Deutsch, M. B., ... Operario, D. (2015). HIV risk and preventive interventions in transgender women sex workers. *The Lancet, 385*(9964), 274–286.

Reisner, S. L., White, J. M., Bradford, J. B., & Mimiaga, M. J. (2014). Transgender health disparities: Comparing full cohort and nested matched-pair study designs in a community health center. *LGBT Health, 1*(3), 177–184.

Ring, D., & Lawn, S. (2019). Stigma perpetuation at the interface of mental health care: A review to compare patient and clinician perspectives of stigma and borderline personality disorder. *Journal of Mental Health*, DOI: 10.1080/09638237.2019.1581337.

Seidemann, R., Duek, O., Jia, R., Levy, I., & Harpaz-Rotem, I. (2021). The reward system and post-traumatic stress disorder: Does trauma affect the way we interact with positive stimuli? *Chronic Stress, 5*, 2470547021996006.

Sevelius, J. M. (2013). Gender affirmation: A framework for conceptualizing risk behavior among transgender women of color. *Sex Roles, 68*(11), 675–689.

Sherman, A. D., Balthazar, M., Klepper, M., Febres-Cordero, S., Valmeekanathan, A., Prakash, D., ... Kelly, U. (2021). Approach and avoidant coping among black transgender women who have experienced violence: A qualitative analysis. *Psychological Services*.

Spencer, C., Mallory, A. B., Cafferky, B. M., Kimmes, J. G., Beck, A. R., & Stith, S. M. (2019). Mental health factors and intimate partner violence perpetration and victimization: A meta-analysis. *Psychology of Violence, 9*(1), 1–17. https://doi.org/10.1037/vio0000156

Sterzing, P. R., Ratliff, G. A., Gartner, R. E., McGeough, B. L., & Johnson, K. C. (2017). Social ecological correlates of polyvictimization among a national sample of transgender, genderqueer, and cisgender sexual minority adolescents. *Child Abuse & Neglect, 67*, 1–12.

Stevens, J. S., & Jovanovic, T. (2019). Role of social cognition in post-traumatic stress disorder: A review and meta-analysis. *Genes, Brain and Behavior, 18*(1), e12518.

Watt, S. O., Tskhay, K. O., & Rule, N. O. (2018). Masculine voices predict well-being in female-to-male transgender individuals. *Archives of Sexual Behavior, 47*(4), 963–972.

Wolfe, D. A. (2018). Why polyvictimization matters. *Journal of Interpersonal Violence, 33*(5), 832–837.

World Health Organization. (2019). *International statistical classification of diseases and related health problems* (11th edition). WHO. https://icd.who.int/

CHAPTER 8

INTRODUCING THE TRIPHASIC MODEL

Let's start with the bad news. There is a strong and growing literature about exposure rates to trauma and stress in a wide range of TGD populations, but a relative dearth of process-based or outcomes-based research. This mirrors gaps in the field overall, as there is a comparative scarcity of research on therapy process or the outcomes associated with clinical work. Process- and outcomes-focused psychotherapy research tends to be time-consuming and expensive to produce, and in order to fit into the model of the scientific method, the treatment itself is generally very tightly controlled. This does not readily lend itself to the somewhat messy and individual work of ongoing psychotherapy. Moreover, while trauma-focused treatments do in fact have some of the most robust process-focused and outcomes-focused research literature in psychology, much of it does not make space for the existence of TGD people, let alone our inclusion.

In some ways, however, this offers more flexibility in considering the breadth of available treatments for the purposes of this manuscript. In the next few chapters, I'll talk about some treatments that have a strong research literature, and also some that have very little published empirical support. As far as I'm concerned, any of them might be helpful for you in how you approach your work with TGD people, because I know that not everything that is helpful has been studied yet, and that not everything that might be helpful lends itself to studies based on the scientific method. Because I know that TGD people have been historically marginalized and understudied by the scientific community, I'm open to the possibility that marginalized and understudied *treatments* could potentially have great value for TGD people, trauma survivors, and TGD trauma survivors. In the course of the next few chapters, I'll lay out the research related to a number of clinical theories and modalities, including some that are less commonly practiced or studied. I'll also talk more about my own approach, which draws from a number of methodologies, and endeavor to illustrate my approach through talking about the case histories. I encourage you to take what works for you and leave the rest. I know that some clinicians prefer to stick with trauma treatments that have a robust research literature. If you feel this way, I encourage you to take this opportunity to interrogate that belief. Do you feel this way because you want to offer the best available treatment to a population that has been underserved and marginalized? Or does it make you uncomfortable to consider ways of offering treatment that are not necessarily rooted in the (white, cisheteronormative, colonial) scientific method? I will acknowledge that I barely have an answer for this for myself, and I don't know what your answer will be, so for now I'll just reiterate that I hope you will work in the way that feels most congruent with your values while also examining those values.

Wherever your clinical values stand, there are a wide variety of ways to formulate and treat the sequelae of trauma and stress. There are cognitive behavioral interventions, psychodynamic interventions, somatic interventions, and interventions that are unique and specific to unique and specific models. Some clinicians find it most effective to start with body-based interventions intended to calm the nervous system. Others prioritize building cognitive control over affect, while still others suggest that beginning with repeated exposure to the stressor has the greatest efficacy. It is my perspective that these debates miss some of the nuance of treatment. For one thing, a fixed position about the "best" treatment for

DOI: 10.4324/9781003140740-9

trauma sequelae misses the unique circumstances that each client represents. An adult who experienced chronic maltreatment as a child might not have specific memories to which to tie imaginal exposure, for instance, which might make methods like prolonged exposure therapy inappropriate for this individual. Someone who developed in a supportive environment and then experienced a terrorist attack as an adult might have a lot of capacity for affective regulation across many domains of experience, but find themselves debilitated by memories of the attack, so starting with skills training in affect regulation might be less helpful for this person. In my experience, ideal treatment modalities vary from client-to-client, and this variation depends on the client's experiences and strengths as well as their freedom to choose the kind of treatment they want. There are data to support this position, including a meta-analysis of the literature related to client choice in therapy (Swift et al., 2018). This meta-analysis found that when clients had choice regarding the types of activities done in therapy, the type of therapy, and goodness-of-fit with the therapist, premature dropout of therapy was reduced by an odds ratio of 1.79. It is my understanding that goodness-of-fit is based partially on variables related to identity and partially on things like personality and therapeutic style. The research suggests that factors like personality fit are more important than identity-matching, but of course personality and therapeutic style are also partially mediated by identity factors. I am not aware of research regarding identity-matching with TGD clients specifically, or literature that indicates whether or not having a TGD clinician enhances treatment outcomes. I imagine this would also be client-specific. Some TGD people really want to work with TGD clinicians. Since most of my clients endorse this as a strong preference, my sample is biased. I also certainly know TGD people who have had excellent therapeutic experiences with cisgender therapists. These identity factors and preferences would likely be something to explore in the treatment itself, and relative to this I think clinicians should work to be open and non-defensive in sharing their social location.

Social location is important, and of course professional location plays a large role here as well. Your training, experience, and competencies play a crucial role in the interventions you select, and whether or not those interventions land as intended. You may feel very competent at acceptance and commitment therapy for trauma and stress, but lost when trying to offer a psychodynamic or relational intervention. In addition to questions of competency, there are also questions of satisfaction—it may be that you would rather claw your eyeballs out than learn somatic methods, for instance. That's perfectly fine—everyone has different eyeballs. Interventions that I find universally useful might not be interesting or effective for you, and vice versa. You get to exercise a lot of choice about the styles of treatment you opt to pursue, and, in many settings, which potential clients you feel equipped and excited to work with. The next several chapters will endeavor to present a fairly high-level overview of some of the more common forms of trauma treatment, as I conceptualize them fitting in to the triphasic model of trauma treatment, and also into the physical, psychological, and interpersonal frameworks discussed in Chapters 5–7. Different clinicians would likely identify different protocols as belonging to different phases or eliminate discussion of some of these treatments altogether while centering others I don't touch on. Let's begin with the overarching framework I employ, which is the triphasic model of trauma treatment.

WHAT IS THE TRIPHASIC MODEL?

The triphasic model of trauma treatment was first outlined by Judith Herman in *Trauma and Recovery: The Aftermath of Violence—From Domestic Abuse to Political Terror* in 1992, and has benefited from many updates and expansions over the intervening decades. The model postulates that, in recovering from trauma, the trauma-exposed person benefits from three phases of treatment: a period of building safety and stabilization, a period of reprocessing the trauma or traumas, and a period of integration or reintegration into a community or communities. Although this is outlined as sequential steps, Herman notes that these phases are not really sequential—a therapeutic dyad may spend some time in the first phase, jump to the third, backtrack to the second briefly before revisiting the first and then again initiating the second. These might, indeed, all happen in the same session. Additionally, not everyone is going to be prepared to go through all of these phases in the time of your therapy. For instance, if you see kids and teens, or you are seeing someone for explicitly short-term treatment for what-ever reason (e.g., you are working in college counseling, VA, or hospital settings with session limits), making some inroads toward safety and stabilization may be the most you can do in a given course of treatment. I would also argue that helping someone build safety and stability is hugely beneficial to their well-being. And, for some people, that work may take months or years to settle. So, if you find that you do a lot of safety and stabilization work, and you also observe that you are seeing the benefits of this work in your clients' lives, please don't feel rushed into reprocessing. While I agree that reprocessing is a very important part of trauma work, I hold the belief that it is most helpful when it comes at the right time, and that it can be harmful when entered into prematurely.

Many of the protocols mentioned below, and described in further detail in Chapters 10–12, don't fit neatly into one of the three phases of the triphasic model (and some of them are explicitly designed to be triphasic, and so could fit into all of the phases). I have made some rather arbitrary distinctions based on my understanding of the primary focus of each model. For instance, cognitive processing therapy does include a period of building safety prior to beginning the written reprocessing, but the focus of the model is on the period of written reprocessing. Skills training in affective and interpersonal regulation incorporates a period of reprocessing, but the focus is on safety and stabilization. In these descriptions, as in treatment and in life, these distinctions are somewhat arbitrary.

PRIMARILY SAFETY-FOCUSED MODALITIES

You may not be surprised to learn that I conceptualize the triphasic model in a way that mirrors the physiological, psychological, and interpersonal chapters of this manuscript. That is to say, when I think about safety, I primarily think about bodily safety, and working on building tools to manage and reduce the effects of physiological hyper- and hypo-arousal.

In my practice, there are two primary goals of the safety and stabilization phase. One part is relative stability in the world. That is, the person has a safe-enough housing situation, a source of income that allows them to purchase food, clothing, medicine, and other necessi-ties, and they are not in a state of active, unmanaged withdrawal from addictive substances. They have any needed mobility or access aids (canes, hearing aids, etc.), and they are not living in conditions where there is active abuse. I feel strongly that clinicians in all settings should work to have knowledge of community-based resources that can help with this kind of assistance, and enough of an understanding of social services to be able to write a letter supporting an application for public housing. This takes on another dimension when work-ing with TGD people, as many community resources and social services organizations are segregated by birth-assigned sex, or by a strictly binary formulation of gender (for instance, a woman might be able to access services if the gender marker on her state ID is M, but a gen-derfluid individual with similar presentation and documentation might not be able to). I will acknowledge that it is deeply frustrating to be involved in these systems. Helping someone access housing, for instance, is time-consuming, draining, and scary—it is truly frightening to acknowledge the lack of resources available to people trying to navigate various systems of oppression. We may feel scared for our clients and scared for ourselves because no matter how buffered we are against the deleterious impact of systemic oppression, no one is truly outside of their grip. (I know this as a part of my own experience from seeing my father, who was white, cisgender, straight, and raised in a middle-class home, slide slowly and then very quickly into becoming an unhoused person.) The theory behind why people need a degree stability in order to work on recovery from the sequelae of exposure to trauma and stress seems fairly clear to me: stress and trauma reactions are intended to keep us alive in traumatic and stressful situations. Working through these reactions when we need them for continued survival is premature. We can offer supportive therapy to clients in very unstable conditions, but it is difficult and potentially dangerous for a person to change when their unsafe conditions remain the same.

The other part of safety and stabilization as I think of it is relative safety in the body. I would define this as the person having some capacity for consciously upregulating or downregulating their emotional responses using strategies like grounding, deep breathing, or physical activity. It also includes some capacity to notice and talk about nervous system activity, which might include the flight/fight/freeze response, sleep cycles, and eating patterns among others.

The different models of treatment we'll talk about in the chapter focused on safety and stabilization include body-based therapies such as somatic experiencing and sensorimotor psychotherapy. This chapter will include a discussion of substance-assisted therapies that might include beta-blockers, tranquilizers, or psychedelics. We'll also cover some more cognitive or mindfulness-based models that have a strong safety and stabilization component, such as seeking safety, and skills training in affective and interpersonal regulation.

PRIMARILY PROCESSING-FOCUSED MODALITIES

At the annual conference for the International Society for Traumatic Stress Studies in 2021, Barbara Rothbaum, the recipient of the society's 2021 lifetime achievement award, described PTSD as a problem of extinction in her keynote presentation on the state of the field. Intrusion, avoidance, and changes in arousal and reactivity are, she reiterated, a perfectly normal response to a traumatic stressor. But, for most people under ordinary circumstances, the reactions to trauma exposure will go through the process of extinction, and trauma reminders will no longer elicit an extreme degree of reactivity. The difference between people who develop PTSD and those who don't, she went on to say, is that the traumatic memories do not go through the typical process of extinction in people who go on to develop PTSD. The solution to this problem of extinction, according to many PTSD researchers, is therapy that focuses on reprocessing the trauma exposure in a specific and stylized way until the person becomes desensitized to the stimulus and extinction occurs. This is part of the philosophy behind the practice of prolonged exposure therapy. Considered the gold standard of reprocessing-focused treatments, the modality of prolonged exposure operates by asking clients to repeat the story of their traumatic event, including a great deal of sensory detail, and stay with the memory until the power of the memory begins to wane. Clients may tell the story several times in a single therapy session and also record it to listen to at home. Recently, some research studies have begun augmenting this reprocessing with virtual reality, for an immersive experience of exposure. Another modality, cognitive processing therapy, operates on a similar principle, but asks participants to write out their traumatic memory rather than telling the story out loud. Eye-movement desensitization and reprocessing has a reprocessing component and also incorporates bi-neural activation (typically in the form of side-to-side eye movement). There are also cognitive behavioral interventions for trauma and PTSD. One of these, the unified protocol, targets symptoms related to minority stress in LGBTQ adults.

We will review these forms of reprocessing, as well as other forms of treatment that have a strong reprocessing component. These include interpersonal therapy, and trauma-informed psychodynamic and eclectic therapies. Psychodynamic reprocessing is the modality I use most frequently. The evidence base for these treatments is geared more toward theory and case history than RCT, so these treatments are sometimes overlooked or under-considered, and we will also touch briefly on some ideas of why this might be the case.

PRIMARILY INTEGRATION-FOCUSED MODELS

I can't overestimate the importance of integration or reintegration into a community for treating the sequelae of trauma and stress in TGD people. Some TGD people who have experienced trauma were members of a strong community prior to coming out, and many lose access to that community support—or access to those communities entirely—as a function of coming out. We know, moreover, that social support is a crucial resilience factor in the wake of trauma exposure, and that people with flexible and meaningful community connections simply do better in recovering from trauma exposure than people without those resources. Until a TGD person has come out, however, their true self may never have never been in community, no matter how close-knit their family of origin, church, or sports team. Additionally, people of all genders who experience childhood maltreatment frequently describe never feeling close or connected to others, as they were asked to carry too many secrets to allow for real intimacy. Gender and sexual minorities who are also survivors of childhood maltreatment carry double the secrets, which can multiply the shame exponentially. Thus, people in this situation may stay away from any kind of community entirely, or only engage with others whom they perceive to be ashamed in the same ways.

Although integration or reintegration into the community can look like a lot of different things, for many TGD people it incorporates an element of advocacy and activism. Many TGD people report feelings of connection and liberation when taking ownership of their identities, and engaging in activism that asserts unequivocally and unapologetically that trans lives matter. There is also an element of growth and development for many TGD people in being fully accepted in their gender by other people with marginalized gender identities, and all working together on something that is bigger than the individual.

In addition to connecting TGD individuals with spaces that focus on activism, other forms of treatment that we'll discuss which center the integration or reintegration phase are relational therapy, acceptance and commitment therapy, and feminist psychotherapy.

MODELS OF TRAUMA TREATMENT
ALONGSIDE MODELS OF GENDER DEVELOPMENT

Although the development of TGD identities in under-researched, there are now a few models of TGD gender development. These include stage-based models (e.g., Bockting & Coleman, 2007; Devor, 2004) as well as those centered around master narratives (e.g., Bradford &

Syed, 2019). My understanding of TGD identity development is tripartite, and in some ways maps on to the physiological, psychological, and environmental chapters of this book. This tripartite model has been formalized in several qualitative research articles, although the language they use is somewhat different from one article to another. One article focuses on providing what the authors call an eco-developmental framework at the intersection of gender identity and sexual identity (Lindley et al., 2021). Through content analysis of interviews with young adult men and masculine-spectrum individuals, this study maps various aspects of gendered development onto the micro, meso, and macro-levels of ecological systems first articulated by Bronfenbrenner (for an overview of the theory and a critique from within a disability studies frame, see Sontag, 1996). These researchers identified embodiment as a micro-level consideration and identified use of the body, effects of the body, and hormone treatment as embodiment concerns in their sample. At the meso-level, this article identified dating, attraction, and partner dynamics as primary considerations. (I would add in considerations related to non-romantic interpersonal relationships, but this article was focused on the intersection of gender and sexual identity and thus focused on romantic and sexual partnerships.) The macro-level reflected considerations of societal acceptance and scrutiny. These researchers also discuss cross-level effects and multi-level interactions.

My perception is that Lindley and colleagues are in dialogue with Kuper et al. (2018), which takes an intersectional lens to questions of what they call intracategorical complexity and intercategorical complexity. Focusing on qualitative interviews with TGD emergent adults, this research used a grounded theory approach to identifying themes of what they call dimensions of gender related to self, intrapersonal-developmental processes, and the middle ground between. Themes related to the dimension of sense of self included the body/ physical self, gender identity, gender expression, and gender presentation. Themes related to intrapersonal-developmental processes included awareness, exploration, meaning-making, and integration.

A similar, grounded theory approach with TGD children and adolescents also described two linked dimensions: an internal/personal dimension and an interactional/social dimension (Pullen Sansfaçon et al., 2020). These researchers identified bodily processes, and particularly gender dysphoria, as personal, and exploration and experimentation as social. They described an additional middle ground of processes that were both personal and social, including meaning-making through interactions with important others.

Although these theoretical formulations have some differences, they also have a great deal of similarity in the identification of several facets as important to the development of a TGD identity. (And, although the stage models and master narrative models have somewhat different framing, they typically identify these elements as well.) The first is recognition that gender is something that is felt internally as part of a sense of embodiment. The second is that gender is also something that happens socially, in how we are taken in and reflected by our larger environment. And the third is that there is the space in between the strictly embodied and the strictly environmental, in the interpersonal, intrapersonal, and combinatorial processes of the meso-level.

As with the triphasic model of trauma treatment, this tripartite model of TGD gender development is not fixed, and there is very little that can be neatly and definitively placed in any one category. But both of these models will provide a framework for formulating and understanding the experiences of trauma-exposed TGD people, as we will explore further in Chapters 10–12.

WORKS CITED

Austin, A. (2016). "There I am": A grounded theory study of young adults navigating a transgender or gender nonconforming identity within a context of oppression and invisibility. *Sex Roles, 75*(5), 215–230.

Bockting, W., & Coleman, E. (2007). Developmental stages of the transgender coming out process: Toward an integrated identity. In: R. Ettner, S. Monstrey, & E. Eylered (Eds), *Principles of transgender medicine and surgery* (Vol. 1, pp. 185–208). The Haworth Press.

Bradford, N. J., & Syed, M. (2019). Transnormativity and transgender identity development: A master narrative approach. *Sex Roles, 81*(5), 306–325.

Devor, A. H. (2004). Witnessing and mirroring: A fourteen stage model of transsexual identity formation. *Journal of Gay & Lesbian Psychotherapy, 8*(1–2), 41–67.

Herman, J. L. (1992). *Trauma and recovery: The aftermath of violence from domestic abuse to political terror.* BasicBooks.

Kuper, L. E., Wright, L., & Mustanski, B. (2018). Gender identity development among transgender and gender nonconforming emerging adults: An intersectional approach. *International Journal of Transgenderism, 19*(4), 436–455.

Lindley, L. M., Nagoshi, J. L., Nagoshi, C. T., Hess III, R., & Boscia, A. (2021). An eco-developmental framework on the intersectionality of gender and sexual identities in transgender individuals. *Psychology & Sexuality, 12*(3), 261–278.

Pullen Sansfaçon, A., Medico, D., Suerich-Gulick, F., & Temple Newhook, J. (2020). "I knew that I wasn't cis, I knew that, but I didn't know exactly": Gender identity development, expression and affirmation in youth who access gender affirming medical care. *International Journal of Transgender Health, 21*(3), 307–320.

Sontag, J. C. (1996). Toward a comprehensive theoretical framework for disability research: Bronfenbrenner revisited. *The Journal of Special Education, 30*(3), 319–344.

Swift, J. K., Callahan, J. L., Cooper, M., & Parkin, S. R. (2018). The impact of accommodating client preference in psychotherapy: A meta-analysis. *Journal of Clinical Psychology, 74*(11), 1924–1937.

CHAPTER 9

PHASE 0: BEFORE GETTING STARTED

As more clinicians and clinical researchers grapple with our own assumptions about gender identity and expression, we become better prepared to serve the TGD people who seek our services. Of course, the need for this kind of education is ongoing. Fortunately, there are several avenues for clinicians to explore, some of which may be familiar to you and some of which may be new. At the time of this writing, for instance, WPATH offers courses (and certification) related to its Global Education Initiative for transgender health education. Becoming a GEI-certified clinician is time-consuming and expensive, as it requires multiple days of classes, ten hours of clinical supervision, and several other components (including being a full member of WPATH, which is associated with an annual fee). At the time of this writing, there is not easy-to-access information about scholarships or low-fee opportunities to pursue this training, although with one component (the supervision hours), there is variability, as the fees are paid directly to the supervisor. (Some supervisors also have sliding scale or group opportunities available.) If you anticipate seeing many TGD people in your practice or want to become more conversant with the diagnostic principles related to gender dysphoria/gender incongruence, it may be worth your while to seek out this training. If you would like additional training regarding writing letters of support, you might take a look at The Gender Affirmative Supportive Surgery Evaluation Tool (Gender ASSET), developed by Colt St. Amand and Bec Sohka Keo, or Moe Ari's Writing Clinical Letters of Referral for Gender Affirming Medical Care. A focus on letters is crucial for mental health providers who are planning to see TGD people, in part because some forms of gender-affirming medical intervention require a letter of support from a behavioral health clinician.

I want to pause for a moment and simply reflect on how non-affirming and even grotesque this model is. Millions of people who have wanted medical treatment for gender incongruence, often people who have struggled mightily against a dominant narrative of gender identity and expression and developed a nuanced and multifaceted understanding of their experiences in the world, have had to submit to interviews from mental health services providers in order to pursue gender-affirming medical interventions. While many of the behavioral health providers they have sought these letters from are kind people who are invested in the health and well-being of their clients, most of these providers have received little or no training in gender development or understanding TGD identities, and many may not have had the opportunity to reflect on their own gender identity and expression, or work through cis-centered biases they may hold. Some providers may truly wish to be TGD-affirming and still have judgments about what it means to be TGD. Indeed, one of the most frequent consultation questions I come across in gender-affirming clinical spaces is a provider feeling that there is "something else going on" and wanting advice for how to slow down the process of their client seeking gender-affirming treatment. That provider's feelings can literally keep a TGD person from accessing life-saving medical treatment. A provider can also insist that the TGD person attend as many sessions as the provider wants before writing a letter or simply refuse to write a letter after many sessions. As far as I am aware, there are no data to indicate the mean number of sessions clinicians require to provide letters of support. Nor has there been any research exploring the relationship between number of pre-letter sessions and client satisfaction with the medical interventions. Finally, as far as

DOI: 10.4324/9781003140740-10

I'm aware, there is no research to indicate whether or not the number of sessions a clinician might require prior to writing a letter varies as a function of systemic oppression. We know that letter access is most certainly impacted by client socioeconomic status, as clinics that offer these letters at low- or no-fee tend to have long waiting lists and only exist in a handful of (generally more expensive overall) urban areas. But how do white supremacy, ableism, and anti-fat bias show up in these spaces?

All of that said, at the time of this writing, access to gender-affirming medical treatment most frequently begins in the offices of mental health clinicians, and letters of support are a common need for TGD people with and without trauma exposure. While the rest of this chapter will focus on other aspects of a TGD-affirming practice, please make sure to seek the training and supervision you need to write these letters. There are samples in the WPATH SOC, as well as online, and some surgeons (and most pediatric gender clinics) will have a specific template they want a provider to follow. Requirements also vary by insurance provider, so you may need to reach out to the provider line of your client's insurance in order to make sure you are providing the information they require. I believe the letter writing process is deeply flawed, and I do not like compromising the confidentiality of the therapy space in order to provide medical information to an insurance adjudicator. However, letters that adhere to current guidelines can make the difference between insurance approval and a length appeals process, so please take it seriously. TGD people deserve to get what we are looking for when we seek treatment. Additionally, if you *are* comfortable writing letters of support for gender-affirming services, and willing to donate some time to TGD people seeking surgery, I encourage you to take a look at the Gender Affirming Letter Access Project, which maintains a registry of providers who are willing to provide pro bono gender assessments and letters of support.

As you move into learning more about writing letters, it may be helpful to bear in mind that the most common co-occurring mental health diagnosis, alongside gender dysphoria/gender incongruence, for people seeking gender-affirming treatment is: no diagnosis. Yep, most of the time people present to clinicians simply because they want a letter of support for hormone treatment or gender-affirming surgery, they have no mental health concerns that meet DSM diagnostic criteria. Now, because I work with trauma, most of the TGD people that I personally work with *do* have mental health concerns and sometimes quite complex biopsychosocial needs. But this is not true for the majority of TGD people seeking letters of support. (For further discussion on the topic of letters, and discussions of the informed consent model of gender-affirmative hormone treatment, see Ashley, 2019; Cavanaugh et al., 2016; Deutsch, 2012.)

Turning toward other ways of practicing gender inclusion in your practice, one place to start is through signifying your gender-affirming intentions in your description of your practice. For instance, if you have a website, Psychology Today profile, or client-facing media, you may want to avoid descriptions such as "I see men, women, and teens…" which excludes people who are neither men nor women and may also leave TGD men and women wondering if they would be welcome. More inclusive language might be along the lines of "I see adults and teens of all genders." You might also choose to state explicitly "I am a gender-affirming therapist." Offering your pronouns in your description of your practice, on your business cards, or in your email signature, is also another small way to indicate allyship.

In addition to descriptions of clients or patients you would welcome, you might also take a look at how you describe your therapy groups and spend some time thinking about how you construct these groups (if you run groups). Affinity groups for members of marginalized communities are an important part of the group landscape, and some of these are segregated by gender and/or sexual identity. Thinking through these kinds of affinity groups can also be the place in which many clinicians start to observe some rigidity or discomfort in their thinking about gender identity and expression. If you are planning, for instance, an LGB women's group, would it be open to a bisexual woman with a beard? Or a genderfluid person who is sometimes a woman? This doesn't mean that you should never have affinity groups based on gender, but you should be clear and intentional about whether or not these groups are trans-affirming, including being prepared to address instances of transphobia that arise in the groups themselves. How will you handle a group member misgendering another group member? How will you handle it if you misgender someone in front of the group? What if someone misgenders you? If you do decide to do gender-based affinity groups, you might consider adding verbiage to indicate that anyone who finds a home in women's spaces/men's spaces is welcome, or adding the trans flag to your materials for the group, or simply stating "all women and feminine-spectrum people are welcome" or "all men and masculine-spectrum people are welcome." You may also choose to have a separate affinity group for TGD people. While this is certainly a worthwhile endeavor, and TGD affinity groups can be very helpful for many TGD people, some of the issues TGD people experience are not related to TGD identity *per se*. The difficulties of a gay man may be more related to his sexual identity, which would make a gay men's group a more appropriate referral for him than a gender exploration group. A nonbinary person of color may benefit more from a group centering BIPOC people of all genders in which they may be the only TGD person than in a group centering TGD people in which they may be the only BIPOC person. A gay autistic TGD BIPOC individual may hate affinity groups and prefer to be in a general support group and may also need some additional support from a facilitator when systemic oppression is enacted in the context of the group space.

If you work primarily or exclusively with children and families, you already know a lot more than I do about navigating family systems in which the children have needs that the parents are struggling to meet. If a family with a TGD or gender-questioning child comes to your practice, what do you see as your role in advocating for the child within the family system? What about within the larger medical system of a pediatric gender clinic? Can you confidently refer to a gender clinic in your area or to a TGD-competent pediatrician? In the United States, people under the age of 18 are not able to access medical treatment without the consent of their guardian, barring a lengthy and uncertain court process (for a discussion of the ethics of this issue, see Dubin et al., 2020). Even *with* the consent of a guardian, these services can be difficult or impossible to access in much of the country. People under 18 are rarely able to access surgery, and never without parental consent. (I hate that I even have to say this, but because contesting this has become a prominent piece of disinformation I'll reiterate: *no-one of the age of 18 can access gender-affirming surgeries without parental consent.* The only exceptions to this have related to intersex children, who have frequently been subjected to genital surgery. This has sometimes happened in infancy or early childhood, without their consent or assent, and sometimes also without parental knowledge or consent.) What if you were to see a family in which one (or both, or all of) the adults were TGD? How would the gender dynamics influence your formulation regarding the health of the family? What if the family were a polycule with many adult members? Or the family were a single parent and child of different races, both of whom were transitioning? Would it be difficult for you to support a person in transition if you were working with them as part of a couple and worried that the transition might mean the demise of the relationship? Might you feel unconsciously pulled to overidentify with the non-transitioning partner? You may not really know the answers to these questions prior to encountering these situations, but spend some time thinking through these permutations and getting very clear in your capacity to work with TGD people in a variety of family constellations.

Assuming that you have thought through your areas of expertise and also your limits, and made your gender-affirming aspirations known in client-facing media, the next piece of your practice that a client would experience might well be related to your intake paperwork. For our purposes, this means the paperwork/electronic paperwork you offer your clients, the system into which you enter client information, and the system you use for insurance billing, even though your clients would likely only see the first of these. The overarching question here that I'll ask you to consider is: why do you need the information you are asking for? It is my opinion that that is the primary question through which to interrogate our paperwork. It may be that gender is not actually relevant to your intake procedure, in which case you may consider deferring the question. You might not need to know someone's gender identity until several sessions have passed, and greater trust has been established. Actually, realistically, you probably *won't* know someone's gender identity until trust has been established, whether you ask the question or not. So, what are you hoping to learn by asking this question in your intake paperwork?

I know that this is controversial, but I want to take the opportunity to pose a separate, but related, question here. Do we need to know about trauma history in the intake paperwork or even in our first sessions? Asking someone to disclose trauma—even a simple, non-detailed disclosure that the person experienced trauma—is a big ask. Answering this question in any kind of meaningful way can really throw off someone's hard-won stability. It may be that this person wants to know more about you, and your ability to tolerate hard things with them, before making this disclosure. I trained in several trauma-specific training programs, and our intake processes almost always included a traumatic experiences interview with a clinician who may or may not be assigned as the interviewee's clinician. (This was frequently linked to funding, and sometimes to determining if the client was "traumatized enough" to receive services.) This is a difficult dialectic for me because most of the time I think clinicians don't ask about and formulate around trauma frequently enough. But if trauma is going to be asked about, it is usually asked about during intake, and I'm not sure this is our best approach. I encourage you to simply consider your values around it. While I learned a lot from conducting these trauma interviews, I'm not sure that it was beneficial, or even neutral, for the people coming into the clinic.

Returning to the question of gender identity, if knowing someone's gender (or at least their first answer to your first question about gender) is important to your practice, you may want to update your paperwork to ask about pronouns and gender identity in an open-ended way (e.g., as a fill-in-the-blank rather than a forced-choice option). If you do use a dropdown list or forced-choice options, avoid listing the options as "woman" "man" "trans woman" and "trans man" because trans women are women and trans men are men. You might consider woman, man, nonbinary, and not listed (with a box to fill in a different gender identification). It might also be helpful to allow a user to select multiple answers.

Think carefully, as well, about asking for someone to identify their sex assigned at birth. Do you work in a medical clinic or in some other space in which this is pertinent information? For instance, we did ask about sex assigned at birth in the psychophysiology lab, in part because some of the safety protocols related to fMRI insist that every AFAB person receive a pregnancy test, whether capable of getting pregnant or not. I would certainly ask if I were doing health-disparities research related to gender, where it might be really important to know if there are health-disparities differences in AMAB nonbinary people and AFAB nonbinary people, for instance. (I would want to know hormone usage status as well, for both trans and cis people.) But do I need to know for the sake of my private practice? Generally not, and if there comes a time when I *do* need this information, it is easy enough to ask about it then. You probably *do* need to know someone's legal name and the gender marker on their identification, if not right away then fairly early, for legal purposes and the purposes of notes and billing. You might also want to clarify if the name and gender marker on their identification is the same name and gender marker their insurance has for them. Many people change their name on their identification years before updating it with their insurance. When asking about names and gender markers, it can be helpful to separate out your questions. You might ask for "name you use/name I should call you" and "name on your state-issued identification," for instance. (Terms of preference, such as "preferred name" and "preferred pronouns" are considered dated and should not be used for these questions.) Just to add another level of complication, someone might have a name that they use that is also their legal name (e.g., has been changed with the court) and still have an old name on their state-issued identification. Think about which of these you really need to know, and ask your questions accordingly. Just as a reminder, even if you know the name on someone's legal identification (sometimes called a "deadname," "birth name," "original name," or "previous name") do not use this if they have asked you to use something else, except under very specific circumstances as described below.

The takeaway here is that, while there may be good reasons to ask about any or all of these signifiers of identity and experience, consider avoiding asking about them without a solid rationale. Also be mindful about sharing your rationale with your clients and letting them know about possible outcomes related to your questions. For instance, suppose you ask for the name and gender marker that is known to their insurance company. Clarify that you will use this information for insurance billing purposes only, and that it means that they will receive information from their insurer in that name (or, if you are providing a superbill, that they will receive a statement from you in that name). If you're asking about someone's pronouns in therapy, you might clarify that you will be writing therapy notes about the sessions, explain that the notes are protected by confidentiality, and ask what pronoun to use in the notes. If you are writing a letter of support for surgery, let them know that you will be parenthetically mentioning the name known to their insurance, but not referring to them by that name, and ask what pronouns they would like you to use for the context of the letter. Same if you'll be talking with a past clinician, or with their psychiatrist or primary care provider. And if you receive a call from, say, an inpatient unit, and the caller is using your client's old name and incorrect pronouns, follow that provider's lead until you are able to talk with your client. Your client may be making a safety choice, and outing them would be a violation of confidentiality as well as their trust. Short version: in working with TGD people and people who have experienced trauma, transparency about your motives, intentions, and the range of possible outcomes, is much preferred to surprises.

After you have made some decisions about your own intake paperwork and thought about the ways in which you want to frame your questions around gender identity and expression, you'll likely need to take a look at your notation system, which is probably some sort of electronic medical record. It is becoming more common for these to have space for the name that someone uses that isn't their legal name (usually designated in these systems as "Preferred Name"). The system I use has a dropdown box for "Legal Gender," but that is the field that populates to CMS forms, so what it really means is insurance gender, unless this person will not be using insurance, in which case it would mean gender marker on state-issued identification. However, some of the options for "Legal Gender" include

"Transgender Male to Female" and "Transgender Female to Male," which are not recognized by either insurance companies or on state or federal identification. Finally, you may want to review the interface between your notations system and whatever larger billing system is in play (e.g., insurance, the veteran's administration, or HMO you work for).

After encountering your paperwork, the next exposure to your practice that your client may have would be exposure to your physical space. When I first started in private practice, I took office space under the assumption that there were single-user bathrooms on every floor of the building. This was not the case—in fact, all of the bathrooms, other than those in a small doctor's office on the first floor that was locked against non-patient entry, were multi-user and gender-segregated. This did give me the opportunity to practice advocacy. First, I spoke with the administrator of the medical practice asking if it would be possible for my clients to use their facilities. She did not feel comfortable with this due to concerns about the privacy of her patients. Then, I spoke with the property manager, requesting that some of the restrooms be designated all gender, or the signage changed to "urinals" and "no urinals," or even that some of the bathrooms be separated into single-user (which would have required constructing an additional wall). The property manager informed me that the building owner believed these changes would be inappropriate because "we see so many families here." Had I been a bit more advanced in my career and had more experience in my role as an advocate, I would have reminded her that TGD people are also members of families, and that many families have TGD members, and that everyone deserves a safe place to pee. While this particular round of advocacy was ineffective, and I did not pursue it to the extent I wish I had, I did notice that the next office building she developed with the same owner *did* have single-user bathrooms. In the meantime, the workaround for the space I was in was to tell prospective clients—all prospective clients—about the set-up prior to our first meeting, and also to direct them to the nearest single-user, gender-inclusive restrooms in the vicinity (in this case it was at a nearby coffee shop).

Ideally, you will find office space that allows you to have single-user, gender-inclusive restrooms that are also truly wheelchair accessible and comfortable for people with a range of body sizes. If that is not available to you, consider advocacy around making multi-user bathrooms more gender-inclusive through changing signage, etc. If that is not feasible for you, look for a safe and useable alternative bathroom in your vicinity, and make sure you let people know about the facilities in advance of their first appointment. Please don't spring a surprise gender-segregated, multi-user restroom on your clients, especially if your building welcomes a mix of TGD and cisgender people. This is psychologically unsafe for your TGD clients and could be physically unsafe for them as well (for a discussion of gender-segregated bathrooms and the effect on TGD youth, see McGuire et al., 2022.)

The next thing to consider is who else might be in your office space and waiting area, which could potentially be a client-facing administrative assistant, other clinicians, the clients of other clinicians, or all of these depending on your set-up. Administrative assistants have a tough job, and frequently do the incredibly important early work of building trust and rapport. If you work in an environment with a client-facing administrative assistant (e.g., a doctor's office or a college counseling center), that person deserves to be trained in gender-affirming practices. They will probably also need some support in changing office practices, as many of these practices may be rooted in past policy or past perceptions of politeness. Support might include reminding them not to use pronouns or gendered honorifics such as Mr. or Ms., and remembering to use the name with which people introduce themselves rather than the name on their documentation. If your office has gender-segregated, multi-user bathrooms that are kept locked, and a client must ask an administrative assistant for keys to access the facilities, it may be simplest to have both sets of keys openly available, and to ask the administrator to provide directions along the lines of "there's a shared restroom with urinals down the hall to the right, and another without urinals up the stairs to the left." If there may be multi-person public conversations among staff (e.g., there are several administrative assistants, or clinicians and administrative assistants who chat in the waiting area) everyone should be trained in the expectations around respectful dialogue, and everyone should feel empowered to, and accountable for, redirecting or shutting down dehumanizing conversations. Finally, you will need to create a culture of accountability by normalizing this person correcting you when you make an error. I mention all of this because I have worked in environments with quite lovely administrative assistants who were not given the training and support they needed to be gender affirming, and I have seen the detrimental effect that this can have on clients.

If you have a shared waiting room, you may want to have a conversation with other clinicians and any other personnel about waiting room policies and procedures. When I was working in an outpatient hospital setting, a client used their gender-neutral last name as their name. However, the administrator and the other clinicians who shared the space would use that person's first name in talking about them (e.g., I might ask "Where's Jay?" and the response might be "Oh, Shirley is with the psychiatrist.") I have also had clients report experiences of being stared at and whispered about by other clients in the waiting room. On the other end of the spectrum, someone I know who works in a gender clinic has found that sometimes excited clients can be overly chatty and affiliative in the waiting room, asking personal questions about gender of other clients who don't want to discuss or disclose. A conversation about waiting room policies that everyone can agree to can help nip these problems in the bud.

If you are currently a student working in a training environment, you may have observed all of these challenges and more at your placement and not have the autonomy or safety you need to be able to intervene. While many training environments are building toward more affirming practices, not all of them are there yet. I urge you to take your safety seriously in these contexts and also to see if there's a way or place in which you can practice advocacy for your TGD clients and staff (and potentially other trainees and potentially yourself). For instance, if you have an individual supervisor on the staff that you like and trust, you might consider bringing the challenges you observe to their attention. You might also consider enlisting your cohort members for support, if that is safe for you. I am perhaps especially sensitive to this consideration because in my training, I had a fellow trainee call one of my clients "crazy" for using contextual pronouns. While I did push back against this ableist and anti-trans formulation, I still wish that I had been more forceful in my response to this misguided individual, who was left with their anti-trans bias and psychological ableism largely unchecked in this instance.

We have considered ways in which an individual who wants to come to your practice might find you, things to address as they are in the process of presenting to your office, and now we can consider your office space itself. I must acknowledge that I first started thinking about this chapter in the pre-COVID era, when telehealth was much less common and those platforms were less robust. Currently, I do not have office space, and have had the opportunity to think about the ways in which meeting virtually is significantly more inclusive. For people who want to experiment with gender in-session, they can do so from the comfort of their own homes, without worrying about transit, bathrooms, waiting rooms, or carrying clothing with them. Telehealth is simpler for most autistic people and allows the option to transition over to typing if someone is less verbal or becomes overwhelmed in session and wants to continue communicating but not talking. Accessing a gender-affirming clinician is easier by telehealth for people who live in rural areas, as well as people who work long hours, or those who can't afford transit. It is also safer for BIPOC clients than visiting an office in a white part of a segregated town or city (and most towns and cities are racially segregated— the variation is largely one of degree). And it can make the difference between access and no access to people who use mobility aids to get around.

There are certainly drawbacks to telehealth, of course. Telehealth presumes that some- one has internet access, for one, and also can find a private space to engage. It can be more difficult to access body-based cues about what a person might be experiencing in a session. Some people need a safe and separate space to be able to disconnect effectively from their day-to-day life and focus on their internal experience. Some trauma survivors need to be able to "leave the bad stuff" in a separate location. There may be fewer distractions in face- to-face office visits. And many clinicians find telehealth uniquely draining, practice in states that restrict the use of telehealth, or simply have a strong clinical preference for face-to-face interactions.

For those times we prefer to have office space, or find that it facilitates the connection with clients, I recommend a look through the literature on office spaces for background on the contributions of design features, such as color and light, on client perceptions of safety and connection (see, e.g., Backhaus, 2008; Jones, 2020). There is also a literature on creating multiculturally appropriate office spaces (see, e.g., Devlin et al., 2013). I think the question of how to create an office environment that is inviting for a range of people, without tokeniz- ing or appropriating cultural signifiers that aren't our own, is a big one and certainly one I wrestle with. But the choices we make to show tacitly that we understand that safety is a consideration can go a long way toward quieting conscious or unconscious worry in our clients, so you may consider adding office décor that is explicitly TGD-affirming. Having reading material in your waiting room, or visible in your office, for instance, that centers TGD experiences can be a useful signifier of inclusion.

Assuming that someone is able to successfully make it to your office door/Zoom room, and they can afford your services or you take their insurance, and you have space in your case load, and all of the other elements that go into to initiating a therapeutic relationship what comes next? Unfortunately, for too many TGD clients, what might come next is a barrage of microaggressions, especially if the person has multiple marginalized identities.

I want to make sure to mention the biggest misstep a clinician can make when having a client disclose a trans identity: trying to stop the person from being TGD. In the 2015 USTS, 20% of respondents asserted that they had this experience with a provider (James et al., 2016). This experience was associated with a 150% increase in history of attempting suicide.

As mentioned in Chapter 4, there is a developing literature regarding the experience of anti-TGD microaggressions enacted by therapists against TGD clients. A qualitative study identified themes of lack of respect for client identity, lack of competency, saliency of iden- tity, and gatekeeping (Morris et al., 2020). Lack of respect for client identity included a general sense of not being believed, being outed by the therapist to family members or administrative staff, misgendering, denial of identity, and sexualization or exotification of TGD bodies. Lack of competency in this study was reflected by the acknowledgment that there simply aren't enough therapists who have received training in gender diversity, along- side "qualified" therapists expressing fixed, dated, or hostile ideas about gender identity and expression. Saliency of identity was thematically identified as an overemphasis on gender, with the provider expressing the belief that everything the client might be experiencing was related to TGD identity or minimization in which TGD identity was underconsidered.

The gatekeeping theme of this study focused on the diagnosis of gender dysphoria/gender incongruence, the accessibility or inaccessibility of letters of support, and outright denial of services. While I believe this study has a lot to teach providers who work with TGD people, I believe that it underestimates the severity of therapeutic microaggressions because the majority of participants in this study were white and middle class, and educated at the level of high school graduation or above. The majority were also seeking treatment specifically for letters of support, so already had some clear sense of their gender and the interventions that would be helpful to them. That said, I strongly recommend a review of this study for clinicians working with TGD individuals.

Another study that focuses on clinician microaggressions in therapy with TGD clients incorporates the important theme of education burdening, as well as themes of gatekeeping, and an array of gender-based themes such as gender narrowing, gender generalizing, gender repairing, and gender pathologizing (Mizock & Lundquist, 2016). Education burdening is the practice of relying on an individual with a marginalized identity for teaching us about that identity instead of taking steps toward educating ourselves and seeking relevant consultation or supervision. For participants in this study, education burdening had the effect of taking them out of the role of client and asking them to instead be a teacher or trainer.

A parallel study, with several of the same authors, identifies themes of *microaffirmation* that TGD clients have received in therapy (Anzani et al., 2019). These included themes such as acknowledging and disrupting cisnormativity and seeing the TGD client's authentic gender. Another important theme was the *absence* of microaggressions, which the authors note may be setting the bar rather low in terms of positivity and affirmation. Seeing clients' authentic gender was the most frequently identified theme, and, I believe, the therapeutic space in which a clinician can offer a tremendous amount of validation and support with very little effort. Believing our clients when they tell us who they are is kind of our jam, yeah?

When we believe people about their own experiences, it becomes easier to advocate on their behalf, which for TGD clients will probably mean tapping into the network of providers in your area who are able to offer competent care. This means getting to know the work of providers in your area who offer treatment specific to gender affirmation, such as endocrinologists, family medicine doctors, or nurse practitioners who can provide hormones for people who want them. It means knowing the surgeons in your area who offer gender-affirming surgeries and doing a deep dive into the critiques of their surgical work or bedside manner that you can likely find online. If you are able to establish rapport with a TGD-affirming medical provider and build personal relationships, this also gives you the opportunity to practice advocacy related to other facets of intersectional identity. For instance, does a urologist you want to refer to have BMI requirements for bottom surgery and a reputation for fat shaming? Has the plastic surgeon in your network had training and experience in facial feminization surgery for BIPOC women and feminine-spectrum people? Is the LGBTQ+ health clinic in your area accessible to people who use mobility aids? How does the pediatric gender clinic in your area make services available to children on public health insurance?

In addition to building out your referral network for services that are specifically gender-affirming, preparing to treat TGD people in your office means building out your referral network to all kinds of providers for health care that is not specific to TGD people. I once, unthinkingly, referred a TGD person who blended to a physical therapist that I had not evaluated for TGD inclusion. While this referral wasn't the disaster it could have been, it was an uncomfortable experience for my client to have a treatment provider's hand on their body and see this provider's growing awareness of my client's trans identity. And while it is true that we cannot protect our clients from every uncomfortable experience, it is also true that it's difficult to let your body relax and be cared for when you are worried about being judged or harassed.

There are also subtler questions of inclusion and who a particular space is designed for. You may know a wonderful and inclusive gynecologist to whom you would happily refer a man, but who works in a clinic named Women's Health Clinic. Or a wonderful mammography clinic in which all of the smocks are pink and the staff refers to patients as "ladies." This is not to say that you could never appropriately refer a TGD person to care in these spaces. But viewing seemingly neutral spaces through a lens that assesses for gender inclusion will help you recognize that ways in which these spaces can get very complicated very quickly for our TGD clients and loved ones.

I hope this has been a helpful overview of things to consider before beginning trauma treatment with TGD people. Thoughtful attention to these issues can be helpful in illuminating our unexplored biases, which I believe is a crucial part of trauma therapy, work with TGD people, and trauma therapy with TGD people.

WORKS CITED

Anzani, A., Morris, E. R., & Galupo, M. P. (2019). From absence of microaggressions to seeing authentic gender: Transgender clients' experiences with microaffirmations in therapy. *Journal of LGBT Issues in Counseling, 13*(4), 258–275.

Ashley, F. (2019). Gatekeeping hormone replacement therapy for transgender patients is dehumanising. *Journal of Medical Ethics, 45*(7), 480–482.

Backhaus, K. L. (2008). *Client and therapist perspectives on the importance of the physical environment of the therapy room: A mixed methods study* (Doctoral dissertation). Texas Woman's University.

Cavanaugh, T., Hopwood, R., & Lambert, C. (2016). Informed consent in the medical care of transgender and gender-nonconforming patients. *AMA Journal of Ethics, 18*(11), 1147–1155.

Deutsch, M. B. (2012). Use of the informed consent model in the provision of cross-sex hormone therapy: A survey of the practices of selected clinics. *International Journal of Transgenderism, 13*(3), 140–146.

Devlin, A. S., Borenstein, B., Finch, C., Hassan, M., Iannotti, E., & Koufopoulos, J. (2013). Multicultural art in the therapy office: Community and student perceptions of the therapist. *Professional Psychology: Research and Practice, 44*(3), 168.

Dubin, S., Lane, M., Morrison, S., Radix, A., Belkind, U., Vercler, C., & Inwards-Breland, D. (2020). Medically assisted gender affirmation: When children and parents disagree. *Journal of Medical Ethics, 46*(5), 295–299.

James, S. E., Herman, J. L., Rankin, S., Keisling, M., Mottet, L., & Anafi, M. (2016). *The report of the 2015 U.S. transgender survey*. National Center for Transgender Equality.

Jones, J. K. (2020). A place for therapy: Clients reflect on their experiences in psychotherapists' offices. *Qualitative Social Work, 19*(3), 406–423.

McGuire, J. K., Okrey Anderson, S., & Michaels, C. (2022). "I don't think you belong in here:" The impact of gender segregated bathrooms on the safety, health, and equality of transgender people. *Journal of Gay & Lesbian Social Services, 34*(1) 40–63.

Mizock, L., & Lundquist, C. (2016). Missteps in psychotherapy with transgender clients: Promoting gender sensitivity in counseling and psychological practice. *Psychology of Sexual Orientation and Gender Diversity, 3*(2), 148.

Morris, E. R., Lindley, L., & Galupo, M. P. (2020). "Better issues to focus on": Transgender microaggressions as ethical violations in therapy. *The Counseling Psychologist, 48*(6), 883–915.

CHAPTER 10

PHASE 1: SAFETY IN AN UNSAFE WORLD

The overarching philosophy that is captured by prioritizing a phase of safety and stabilization is that the capacity to self-regulate—and particularly to self-regulate through embodiment—is a fundamental component of trauma recovery. This idea is certainly not unique to trauma-oriented therapy, psychotherapy, or the Western European and colonial traditions on which psychotherapy is built. Dance is a practice for trauma recovery and community-building across much of Africa and the African diaspora (see Monteiro & Wall, 2011). Dance has been used quasi-experimentally with Africans who have been displaced from their homes due to natural disaster (Salihu et al., 2021), and in combination with psychoeducation regarding Post Traumatic Slave Syndrome with Black adolescents in Chicago (Campbell, 2019). Mindfulness practices constitute a large part of the safety and stabilization components of trauma treatment modalities such as seeking safety and skills training in affective and interpersonal therapy (STAIR), and these mindfulness practices are taken from—and often a distortion of—Buddhist practices (Grossman & van Dam, 2011). And, of course, trauma-informed yoga is a method for unifying movement and breath that has been practiced as a part of Hinduism for quite some time. Body-based practices for emotion regulation and cognitive practices that center bodily awareness are, in my opinion, an integral part of trauma recovery, and they are not new or unique to our discipline. In fact, many of these practices have been stripped away from their original practitioners by colonialism and are now simply being offered back in new, often decontextualized, formats, and often at the exclusion of the communities who originated the practices.

REVISITING THE WINDOW OF TOLERANCE

Within the framework outlined in this manuscript, in working toward safety and stabilization as the initial focus of treatment, I operate theoretically from the window of tolerance model introduced in Chapter 5. Helping someone understand the trauma response cycle and find strategies for spending more time in the window of tolerance is, I believe, innately useful as a goal in itself. It is also my clinical judgment that this prepares people who have experienced trauma and stress for the reprocessing phase of trauma treatment. It is my bias—and also has been my clinical experience—that expanding an individual's capacity to stay in the window of tolerance most of the time—including during reprocessing—makes the reprocessing both easier and more effective.

SAFETY AND THE TGD BODY

There may be times (and for some people this is *all the time*) in which the world around us is hostile, unsafe, and harmful. We will not always be able to dodge the slings and arrows of such a world. Additionally, as previously discussed at great length, the world, the country, and the therapy office are empirically less safe for TGD people than for cisgender people. Thus, TGD people may have an uneasy relationship with the idea that something might be "safe," or even "safe enough."

DOI: 10.4324/9781003140740-11

Specifically, the world is less safe for TGD *bodies*, and this is especially true for TGD people whose bodies are stigmatized in multiple ways. I can't overstate how important it is to have the capacity to use our bodies for emotion regulation—to have our bodies be safe-enough spaces. Using our bodies for emotional regulation ultimately allows humans to feel safe enough to digest our food, sleep, differentiate between pleasure and pain, and focus our attention. TGD bodies, BIPOC bodies, disabled bodies, fat bodies, and queer bodies are devalued socially, and often devalued by the very inhabitants of those body. Moreover, when we as humans have experienced trauma and stress, our capacity to use our bodies for emotion regulation frequently becomes diminished. This is a real tragedy, as it is when we have had traumatic and stressful experiences that we need our bodies the most. Embodied safety is most important to those who may have the least access to it.

That said, embodiment practices are not new to queer epistemologies any more than they are to other traditions. Queer forms of resistance hold lots of space for radical self-love and include joy and sex as modes of both power and resilience. Although TGD people may have particularly contested relationships with environmental and physiological safety, we also have a long history of resilience through bodily autonomy and pride (see Matsuno & Israel, 2018; this study will also be revisited in Chapter 12).

The body as resource also fits with the models of TGD gender development discussed in Chapter 8. Most TGD people must ultimately find a way to come to terms with a body that reads differently, on a gendered level, than the bodies of cisgender people. This can take some navigation and experimentation, as many TGD people have received messages over many years about the incongruence of their bodies with their gender and have sometimes been told that they simply can't be the gender they are in the bodies they have. Thus, a sense of profound bodily alienation is not an uncommon occurrence in TGD people, even in TGD people with little or no exposure to trauma and stress. I have encountered TGD people without exposure to significant trauma or stress describe themselves as "floating heads," or describing their genitals as "dead zones." TGD gender development begins, the models of TGD gender development agree, with the embodied self as a primary site of gendered inquiry. When TGD people are also seeking treatment for symptoms related to trauma and stress exposure, some of this grappling with embodiment as a gendered phenomenon may occur during treatment, as embodiment goals related to trauma sequelae can underscore questions related to—or discomfort around—gendered embodiment. Meeting your client where they are in terms of a gendered exploration of embodiment is a key element of all therapy with TGD individuals and may be particularly salient in the safety and stabilization phase of trauma treatment. It can also be helpful to keep in mind that sometimes, although not always, medical transition *is* the individual's embodiment goal, and an embodied sense of safety will be very, very difficult to achieve without access to gender-affirming medical interventions.

BODY-BASED TREATMENTS

There are several body-based therapies intended to build safety as part of the treatment of trauma and stress. Although they are all a bit different from one another, the focus of all of them is on learning to regulate nervous system activation in order to help an individual use their body as a place of refuge. Some of these are sensorimotor psychotherapy (SP), somatic experiencing (SE), and trauma-informed yoga. I want to acknowledge from the start that these treatments have less outcomes data than some other forms of treatment; that said, I find some techniques from these modalities extremely clinically useful.

Interventions in any of these domains may include techniques like grounding and visualization, breathing exercises, some form of movement, and sometimes therapeutic touch or self-touch. They all also have an element of mindfulness. SE invites the client to build awareness of physical sensation and then discharge physiological dysregulation related to trauma through using this awareness to move back and forth between dysregulated and re-regulated physical states (for an overview of the theory of SE as well as a cisgender case study, see Payne et al., 2015). A review of SE acknowledged that the peer-reviewed literature is sparse, but noted that that the studies reviewed indicated support for SE for PTSD (Kuhfuß et al., 2021). This review also notes cross-cultural applicability as a strength of the modality.

SP may include elements of pushing or pulling or squeezing objects or wrapping oneself tightly in a blanket or spending time under a weighted blanket (for a conceptual overview of SP that includes a cisgender case history, see Ogden, 2020). One study found that a 12-week course of group treatment with SP significantly reduced the cisgender participants' symptoms of depression and their perceptions of the impact of traumatic events on their lives (Gene-Cos et al., 2016). A study of an adaptation of SP found that, after 20 weeks of group-based treatment that focused on psychoeducation and physiological self-regulation, cisgender participants reported a statistically significant ability to self-soothe as well as decreased anxiety and increased bodily awareness (Classen et al., 2021). However, there was not an overall reduction of PTSD-specific symptoms or dissociation.

A review of yoga for treating symptoms related to trauma exposure found that the studies reviewed indicated a reduction in PTSD symptoms, and that there was a large effect size of yoga on PTSD symptoms (Nguyen-Feng et al., 2019). There was a medium effect size of yoga on symptoms of depression and on symptoms of anxiety.

Regarding studies in these modalities that either centered or included TGD participants, a pilot study of SE for TGD people found a statistically significant increase in psychological quality of life following ten sessions of a group-based intervention modeled on SE (Briggs et al., 2018). An evaluation of trauma-informed yoga for vulnerable populations (which included a handful of TGD participants) reported that participants reported greater capacity for self-regulation and an increased sense of calm after participating in the intervention (Tibbitts et al., 2021). The authors also noted that participants described yoga as helpful for reducing substance use or maintaining sobriety.

MEDICATION-ASSISTED THERAPIES

Psychedelic-assisted trauma therapy, and specifically MDMA-assisted psychotherapy for PTSD, is currently enjoying a surge in popularity. There are a number of research clinics engaged in Phase 3 clinical trials of this modality, and a recent article relates the methodology and outcomes data from the Phase 2 trials (see Mithoefer et al., 2019). The model presented in the study itself follows a triphasic approach, in that the model includes some non-medicated preliminary sessions in which the participant and the researcher-clinicians get to know one another, followed by a session of MDMA-assisted psychotherapy, followed by several non-medicated sessions focused on integrating the experiences of the medication-assisted session. This will then typically include another two MDMA-assisted sessions, each followed by integration sessions. I place this type of treatment in the section on safety, however, because I think that is what the MDMA ultimately offers—it allows the individual the opportunity to feel very safe and connected very quickly, thereby dramatically lowering the stakes on the reprocessing of whatever traumatic material may emerge. (Other clinicians might put this treatment in a reprocessing-focused section, as many people do engage in significant reprocessing while medicated. However, reprocessing is not the focus of the treatment, and the treatment is not considered a failure if no reprocessing occurs.)

The data regarding MDMA-assisted psychotherapy are very strong. This type of treatment can significantly reduce the symptoms of PTSD and has a very limited risk profile in terms of physical risk from the MDMA itself. There is also data to suggest that this type of treatment can be useful outside of the context of the clinic (see Healy et al., 2021). I found the data compelling enough that I obtained certification in the use of MDMA-assisted psychotherapy, although I have not completed the requisite supervised hours to administer this treatment myself, for a number of reasons including that it is time-consuming and currently only taking place in a very limited number of contexts. I want to be clear that I think it is very promising.

I also believe that there are also some areas of concern. Partly this concern relates to a more general problem of mostly white, cisheteronormative researchers decontextualizing Indigenous (and sometimes queer) healing practices and marketing them back to other white, cisgender, heterosexual people. The problem of this is compounded when we think more broadly about the ways in which BIPOC have been punished and imprisoned for these very practices. Additionally, MDMA-assisted therapy itself, as it is practiced in contemporary Northern American and European contexts, is predicated on an explicitly cisheteronormative model: that of a cisgender man and cisgender woman as the treatment team, originally intended to stand in for the parents in a (nuclear) family as well as reduce risk of sexual impropriety with a medicated patient. Finally, my impression of the training as it stands now is that the trainers are not well-equipped to help trainees come to terms with complex questions about power and vulnerability in the treatment space. I hope that the training continues to develop and that access to (safe) training for queer and trans BIPOC providers will be greatly expanded. Until then, I worry about the practice of administering medication that has the capacity to make a person *feel* very safe in a context where unexamined power dynamics may confer a great deal of psychological risk. Other people, including individuals seeking this treatment, may make a very different determination, and I respect that as well.

Other medication-assisted therapies for PTSD include ketamine-assisted therapy, psylocibin-assisted therapy, and therapy that includes the administration of a beta-blocker. Cannabis is also considered treatment for PTSD, and most states that allow the use of medical marijuana list PTSD as a condition that allows for its prescription. Of these medication-based options, the use of beta-blockers seems to have a purely physiological effect. (Beta-blockers keep the individual's heart rate in a narrow range, short-circuiting the body's sympathetic nervous system response; for a discussion of beta-blockers in PTSD, see Giustino et al., 2016.) I have had clients who have used all of these substances, both in and out of clinical settings, to help manage symptoms related to trauma exposure. Some of them have experienced great success, while for others the experience has been more equivocal. All in all, I think these are all promising directions and encourage clinicians to be prepared to have informed and nonjudgmental conversations about these options.

SEEKING SAFETY

Seeking safety is a time-limited, manualized treatment for co-occurring PTSD and substance use and can be used in a group format or in individual therapy. The treatment manual is centered around 25 treatment topics and includes some psychoeducation and some techniques for tolerating and/or alleviating distress (Najavits, 2002). Originally designed for, and evaluated in, cisgender women (Najavits et al., 1998), the majority of the research to-date continues to be studies of cisgender women. Seeking safety generally has a low dropout rate, and a meta-analysis of seeking safety studies found that it is associated with decreases in PTSD symptoms and substance use, although the substance use reductions were less compelling than the reductions in PTSD symptoms (Lenz et al., 2016). This meta-analytic review also found that the effect sizes tended to be larger in studies that were either predominantly white or entirely BIPOC, suggesting that there is an in-group cultural component to the phenomenon of safety.

In terms of the cultural component of TGD representation, seeking safety has been evaluated in women living with HIV, and this study found a reduction in both PTSD symptoms and substance use (Empson et al., 2017). Seeking safety was also evaluated in BIPOC women in Los Angeles, and this study found a reduction in depression, anxiety, and substance use (Takahashi et al., 2021).

I have used seeking safety in group settings ranging from outpatient hospital programs to college counseling and find it a useful and effective access point for treating symptoms arising from exposure to trauma and stress. One of the things I like most about it is that it has a strong case management component right at the beginning. There is an understanding and acknowledgment of the fact that we are not able to seek psychological safety if our basic needs for housing, food, medical care, and transportation are not met, and it makes working on these tasks with our clients a part of treatment.

SKILLS TRAINING IN AFFECTIVE AND INTERPERSONAL REGULATION AND DIALECTICAL BEHAVIORAL THERAPY

Another broadly studied, manualized, phase-based intervention for PTSD is skills training in affective and interpersonal regulation (STAIR). The complete STAIR protocol generally includes an element of prolonged exposure therapy, which will be discussed in greater detail in Chapter 11. However, the first phase of STAIR consists of teaching coping and distress tolerance skills, generally in a group setting. Topics include labeling, managing, and accepting strong feelings, including strong positive feelings. A study of STAIR for cisgender survivors of childhood maltreatment found that individuals who utilized this treatment reported improvements in self-regulation and decreases in PTSD symptoms (Cloitre et al., 2002). A more recent study of a cisgender US veteran population compared five sessions of STAIR against treatment as usual for either PTSD or depression (Jain et al., 2020). Individuals who received five sessions of STAIR reported improvements in social functioning, emotion regulation, PTSD, and depression, while the treatment as usual group did not. Moreover, the effect sizes of these changes ranged from moderate to large.

While a couple of studies using the STAIR protocol mention TGD participants, it is difficult to properly evaluate efficacy for TGD people as the sample sizes are low (e.g., Gudiño et al., 2014).

STAIR was adapted from techniques used in dialectical behavioral therapy (DBT), which is sometimes used in the context of intensive treatments for PTSD and other trauma-related concerns. DBT was developed originally, however, for people with border-line personality disorder. As we reviewed in Chapter 6, most people who are diagnosed with BPD have a history of trauma exposure, and many people with trauma exposure meet criteria for BPD. Marsha Linehan, the creator of DBT, refers to the invalidating environment as the social contributor to BPD, and this invalidation may exist alongside other forms of exposure to trauma and stress, or independently (see Linehan, 1987, for the original formulation, and Linehan, 2020, for the updated and expanded model). One study of DBT for PTSD compares the efficacy of DBT to that of cognitive processing therapy (CPT; discussed in Chapter 11) for PTSD related to child abuse (Bohus et al., 2020). This study utilized data from cisgender women presenting to outpatient clinics in Germany. It found that, while both methods were effective for reducing the symptoms of PTSD, the DBT model evidenced greater efficacy. Additionally, members of the DBT treatment condition were less likely to leave treatment early.

I mention DBT here in part because of a theoretical model that makes the argument that cisnormative social expectations create an intrinsically invalidating environment for TGD people (Sloan et al., 2017). Thus, the treatment model for working with BPD may be well-suited to the treatment of distress, including trauma-related distress, in TGD individuals. The researchers differentiate between clinical distress in TGD people and BPD *per se*, specifying emotion dysregulation as the target for treatment.

ECLECTIC STRATEGIES AND CLINICAL DECISION-MAKING

Because I base my *in vivo* decision-making about interventions on the window of tolerance hypothesis, I will often pull from all of the modalities described above depending on what I perceive to be happening for my client at any given moment, and none of the interventions below is unique to my practice by any means. The first assessment for intervention is whether it seems the person is currently parasympathetic- or sympathetic-dominant. I evaluate this in three ways. The first is observational. When someone trails off, grinds to a halt, or otherwise starts to lose words, I tend to think this is an issue of parasympathetic dominance, and in these situations, I'll typically start with something upregulating. When someone starts speaking very quickly, or making rapid repetitive movements, or is sweaty or flushed for no evident, extrinsic reason, I tend to think this is an issue of sympathetic dominance, and in these situations, I'll typically start with something downregulating.

A second form of assessment is asking the client directly what they think might be helpful, once we have established a shared language for various techniques. I tend to do at least a bit of psychoeducation early on, and this includes talking about various forms of grounding or regulation we might be using. After we've had that conversation, I'll typically frame techniques in an invitational "do you think we should try…?" way, unless someone is clearly in so much distress that they will not be able to respond. If they agree, we'll try a technique, and after we try it out, I'll ask "do you feel better, worse, or about the same?" If the answer is "better" or "the same," we might try a similar technique although perhaps of greater or lesser intensity. If the answer is "worse," we'll likely go from upregulating to downregulating or vice versa. If someone does not respond at all to an invitation to try a technique, it's generally because they are spinning out and starting to lose track of when and where they are.

In those situations, I find that saying their name loudly enough to attract their attention and then just starting a visible technique (shaking out my hands, for instance) can be a helpful intervention.

Low-intensity upregulating techniques I use are shaking out our hands and feet, stretching (whether standing up or sitting down), or smelling an essential oil or something with a strong (hopefully pleasant) scent. Low-intensity downregulating strategies might be breathing exercises, physical grounding ("tell me three green things that you can see"), or a body scan. If someone needs a lot of downregulating very quickly (i.e., they seem to be on the brink of a panic attack or flashback), a brief burst of jumping jacks (if they are able) will bring their heart rate up, thereby activating all of the homeodynamic elements of heart rate reduction when they stop jumping. Another option is stimulating the dive reflex, which is sometimes used as emergency medicine for tachycardia (for a review, see Smith et al., 2012). The dive reflex is activated by the application of cold and pressure to the center of the forehead (an ice cube will generally suffice) as the person leans forward while holding their breath. Actually, I have found that any kind of change in temperature (holding an ice cube, holding something warming) can be helpful for both upregulating and downregulating. Another strategy that seems useful for both upregulating and downregulating is dyadic co-regulation such as tossing a (soft!) ball back and forth.

The third form of assessment I use is my own bodily sensations. Typically when we are in relationship with others and our own bodies are well-regulated, we tend toward co-regulation. By this I mean that if my body perceives that someone is moving into a sympathetic-dominant state, it might move into a parasympathetic-dominant state in a physiological effort to calm and contain. This is very clear with a caregiver and an infant—if the baby starts crying and screaming and the caregiver has a matching reaction (they also start crying and screaming, for instance), the infant will not regulate. If the caregiver offers calm reassurance and tends to the physical comfort of the infant, the infant will usually regulate (many, many new caregivers everywhere would like to remind me that this is not always the case). However, there are also times in which someone's sympathetic or parasympathetic activation is so strong that our bodies begin to match theirs. So, if I am feeling a little numb or disconnected, for instance, I don't necessarily know if the person across from me is feeling overactivated or underactivated. However, a strong awareness of my own sensations provides valuable clinical information and a starting point from which to ask some questions about regulation. Often, these questions will start with "how are you feeling right now?" and sometimes move into "have you had enough food/water/sleep?" questions from there.

CASE HISTORIES

In Chapter 5, I described my initial assessment of Advika as someone who was generally on the parasympathetic-dominant (low) side of the window of tolerance. She reported significant symptoms of dissociation in the form of derealization and depersonalization, including feeling that she was watching her body from the outside, and not noticing when she was hot or cold or hungry or fatigued. My first indicator of this in our therapy time was the way in which Advika would frequently drift off in mid-sentence, sometimes picking the topic up again in a different way, but often drifting to a new topic without seeming to recognize the change. They also described "forgetting" to eat and sleep, perhaps partially attributable to an overreliance on stimulant medication which they described as having no effect on their wakefulness or mood. In terms of formulating her embodied relationship with her gender, it seemed to me that she was at the very beginning of building her embodied sense of gender, and that this process had gotten derailed by early experience.

In thinking about safety and stabilization session with Advika, I first asked about general living conditions. Advika had a steady job, adequate income, and was safe at home. They worked many, many hours, and the rest of their time was generally taken up with family of origin concerns. These factors taken together with depersonalization meant that it had been some time since even things like doctor's visits and dental work had been a priority. Indeed, Advika almost seemed to exist in a fog or a haze outside of work, and it was initially difficult to clarify treatment goals with her.

In terms of navigating differences in our identities, a particular instance stands out in my mind as a time in which I unconsciously centered whiteness, and particularly a white American perspective, although I'm sure this happened more frequently than I realized. This would be when I asked if she thought she'd be interested in a trauma-informed yoga class being offered at a nearby studio, handing her the postcard advertisement which featured a picture of a room full of white cisgender women in a popular yoga pose. "I'm Hindu and from India," they replied, coolly handing me back the ad. "I'm all good on white woman yoga, thanks." I'm sure I blushed to the tips of my (already very pink) ears before I apologized for my carelessness and asked if she'd be open to talking about microaggressions she had experienced with me and in the United States as a BIPOC immigrant. The rupture and repair process around this experience was uncomfortable, which we were able to acknowledge together. Not foreclosing on it, though, made space for them to talk about experiences of microaggressions both between us and outside of the office, and also their growing awareness of the strong desire to pursue training in a form of dance they had learned as a child. The style of dancing she wanted to learn was strongly gendered, so she wasn't sure she would be able to find someone to teach her the woman's dances *and* she was unsure if she would be able to find adequate instruction in the United States. Their desire to revisit dance broadened our conversations about culture, embodiment, and gender, and they were very insightful in describing ways in which they had purposefully disconnected from bodily sensations and awareness as a way to manage gender incongruence, experiences of aggression, and identity-based shame.

In the therapy space, sensory physical grounding such as smelling essential oils or naming five things she could see were most helpful for managing her experiences of numbing out. At the beginning of treatment, Advika would drift off in the middle of almost every sentence, when we talked about gender it was more like multiple times every sentence. So the safety and stabilization phase of our work largely consisted of me gently inviting them back to their body over and over again, without rushing or pushing. In this phase, Advika would reference past trauma casually neither particularly avoiding it nor particularly delving into it.

Daniel was pretty consistently on the sympathetic-dominant (high) end of the window of tolerance, as we were able to confirm through his use of wearable technology. I'm not sure that this would have been apparent from my observation alone, at least not early on, as he was typically measured and precise in his language and I did not see him visibly rattled or flustered for quite some time. I may have been able to deduce it from his alcohol use, which is often an indicator of sympathetic dominance, and from his startle reflex, which I observed one day when someone in a neighboring office bumped the adjoining wall with a loud bang. I could also have assessed him as sympathetic-dominant based on his self-report of anxiety and insomnia. Understanding his embodied relationship with his gender was fairly unequivocal. Daniel knew what he wanted for his body, although this desire was more aesthetic than felt. He wanted to "look like" a man—he already experienced himself as a man. His struggles with embodiment were more around his sexual identity, or perhaps with his gender in sexual relationships, than with his gender as he felt it. He did describe sometimes being surprised that his chest wasn't flat, but once he had top surgery he rarely mentioned his chest at all—it quickly felt to him as if he had always had a flat chest.

In terms of safety and stabilization, Daniel also had an adequate income and was safe at home. He was somewhat unmoored when he first separated from the military, but as soon as he felt he was able to blend, and had the opportunity to change his name and gender marker, he began working in a typically male-dominated field with several other veterans. His alcohol use was high, although in the normal range for a veteran, which made it difficult for him to assess whether reducing his alcohol use was a goal (or, as he put it, if his drinking was "really a problem"). He described wanting to get better sleep, feel less anxious, and maybe cut down on his alcohol use. He also worried about his blood pressure, which he regularly monitored at home, and felt might be elevated due to stress. He did not have a primary care provider, and one of my goals for our treatment was to encourage him to pursue medical management of his blood pressure, especially given a family history of heart attack and stroke.

Because Daniel was quite data-driven, we started with cognitive and behavioral interventions for relieving stress, including use of a sleep diary app, tracking his drinking, and some paced breathing exercises for bringing down stress. In one of our first sessions, I explained respiratory sinus arrhythmia to him and demonstrated that he had the capacity to regulate his own RSA. First, I asked him to find the pulse in his wrist with his fingers. Then I asked him to turn his attention to the fact that his pulse sped up on inhalation and slowed with exhalation. I explained that this difference was a sign of a healthy nervous system, and the bigger the difference between his pulse at inhalation and his pulse at exhalation, the healthier his system. Then we worked on increasing that difference (the ratio of that difference is RSA). For Daniel, as for most people, the easiest way for him to increase his RSA was for him to slow down his exhale, and he found a pattern of breathing (in for a count of four and out for a count of eight) that worked for him. And he did notice that focusing on his breathing while self-monitoring his RSA did help him feel calmer, most of the time. One day, however, Daniel came to my office in a state of near panic. He had gone to the pharmacy prior to coming into my office building, and had been "clocked" and misgendered publicly by a former acquaintance while in the pharmacy. He noticed his heart rate immediately escalated and kept climbing, and his attempts to practice paced breathing in my waiting room had not yielded results. On ushering him into my office, I encouraged him to do a series of jumping jacks, but he felt too self-conscious as he had not yet had top surgery and he was anxious that I would see the way his chest moved and be disgusted by him. Instead, we grabbed a reusable ice pack which he pressed against his forehead, and while he was still anxious and upset, this intervention helped him avert full-blown panic.

It was in that session that I became aware of how much code-switching Daniel engaged in during our sessions, as this was the first time I heard him use African American Vernacular English (AAVE). Initially, I had the feeling that his use of AAVE indicated that he was feeling somewhat safer and more comfortable with me and with the process of therapy. But later, I thought about the kind of safety that code-switching offered him in the context of white supremacy and specifically in the context of my whiteness. (As intersectional fat activist and equity consultant Tigress Osborn put it, when he used AAVE with me he may have been caught off guard rather than being ready to let his guard down.) Another embodied way in which I missed Daniel was around our differences related to the gender binary. Daniel was a man who happened to be of transgender experience. Growing facial hair, monitoring his changing voice, and seeing shifts in his body composition were coming home for him, and he had no ambivalence about transition or desire to unpack or problematize it. I realized I had been inattentive to this aspect of his identity when I asked him one day about pronouns he wanted me to use when coordinating care with his hormone provider. "He. Always he. OK?" he responded tightly. "OK," I replied neutrally. "And I'm sorry I haven't heard what you were telling me about pronouns." He seemed to drop a bit of tension I hadn't been aware he was carrying, and this opened up the opportunity for him to talk about ways in which he was feeling invalidated in his masculinity, especially in his dating life. Daniel was a gay man and interested in dating other gay men. He was already frequently eliminated as a potential dating partner by many men as a function of white supremacy and colorism. Men that did respond to his dating profiles typically led with questions about the size of his dick, which elicited feelings of shame about his gender and incongruence around his genitals. This also brought up a whole slew of feelings related to sex, which we'll also discuss more in the next chapter.

Shai bounced back and forth between sympathetic dominance and parasympathetic dominance, and when we first met, they would flip from hypervigilant and activated to checked out and numb several times in the same session. Their body was simply chronically dysregulated and always preparing for the worst. This kept them trapped in those worst moments of their experience, and the worst moments of Shai's experience were quite, quite terrible. Their bodily cycles showed this dysregulation in many ways. Shai would sometimes go for days without sleeping and then sleep for 16 hours. This sometimes had the effect of shifting their sleep cycle, so then they would spend a month or two as largely nocturnal. This was also how they tended to eat, sometimes actively or passively restricting, and sometimes ravenously. Finally, this kind of cycling was also apparent with how the sensory component of autism manifested for them—sometimes they seemed almost impervious to sensory input, even quite intense sensory input. At other times, small changes in noise levels or lighting were very overwhelming. Shai's relationship with embodied elements of their gender held similar levels, contradictions, and diffuse elements of self-knowledge. They maintained that they had no gender incongruence and were perfectly happy with their body as it was. Over time, they disclosed that they had at one point passively considered bottom surgery, but that they did not think they would ever be able to access this without hormone replacement therapy, which they did not want. Later still, they disclosed that sometimes they desperately wanted bottom surgery, they did not believe they would ever be able to access this due to anti-fat bias among surgeons. All of these things were simultaneously true—they wanted, were indifferent to, and did not want this intervention all in the same mix.

One of Shai's strategies for dissociation was a sadomasochistic retelling of traumatic experiences. In our first session, they almost immediately began talking about being assaulted by two men when discovered sleeping on a roof. This information was related in a very flat and factual tone, almost a mechanical recitation, and I soon interrupted them with my usual spiel about trauma narratives. "I think what you're saying is really important, and I don't want to cut you off." I then pause and monitor the person's facial reaction. In Shai's case, they looked affronted, although sometimes people look scared, or ashamed, or saddened. "At some point I think it will be really important for us to talk about the things that have happened to you, but you don't know me very well yet. I think I can be most helpful to you if you feel really safe and comfortable with me before we move into that part of our work." "What are we supposed to talk about then?" they replied. "Well, why don't we start with how your body is feeling right now." "My *body*? My body feels like shit. How is that interesting?" "Let me be a little more specific. Can you feel your hands and feet right now?" "No. Why, am I supposed to?"

Body scans, progressive muscle relaxation, and co-regulation through throwing a ball back and forth were the primary in-session tools of our safety and stabilization work. Working with Shai also entailed a fair amount of case management, including helping them access benefits, and coordinating with past care providers from the juvenile shelter system. Shai was not safe at home and did not have adequate income, so we also did a lot of safety-planning, and talked about their participation in the informal economy from a harm reduction perspective. This is probably the place in which I was most misattuned to Shai's safety. They were poor in a way that meant missing out on some work could be the difference between eating food from the grocery store and food from a trash can. I was not aware of moral judgment within myself related to sex work, although I probably did have some of that lingering. But I did worry about the risks they sometimes took, around both sex work and using and selling drugs, and this probably made me less effective at really seeing the grueling effect of capitalism on their life, as well as my own, sometimes actively offensive, lack of recognition about the profound luxury of being able to make safer choices.

IN SUM

I hope that the data and case studies together help clarify why I think the safety and stabilization phase is important and illustrate why I reach for the kinds of interventions I do. This will vary, of course, from clinician-to-clinician and client-to-client, but my hope is that you might find some things in this chapter useful for guiding or expanding your thinking about safety and stabilization, or that there may be modalities you read about here that you would be interested in exploring more. As we move into talking about the reprocessing phase, just remember that safety and stabilization never stops. It will be more or less a prominent consideration at different times in your work with a given individual, but we can all get jarred out of the window of tolerance, and finding a way into it, or back to it, is (in my opinion) a crucial part of the work of therapy.

WORKS CITED

Bohus, M., Kleindienst, N., Hahn, C., Müller-Engelmann, M., Ludäscher, P., Steil, R., ... Priebe, K. (2020). Dialectical behavior therapy for posttraumatic stress disorder (DBT-PTSD) compared with cognitive processing therapy (CPT) in complex presentations of PTSD in women survivors of childhood abuse: A randomized clinical trial. *JAMA Psychiatry*, *77*(12), 1235–1245.

Briggs, P. C., Hayes, S., & Changaris, M. (2018). Somatic experiencing® informed therapeutic group for the care and treatment of biopsychosocial effects upon a gender diverse identity. *Frontiers in Psychiatry*, *9*, 53.

Campbell, B. (2019). Past, present, future: A program development project exploring post traumatic slave syndrome (PTSS) using experiential education and dance/movement therapy informed approaches. *American Journal of Dance Therapy*, *41*(2), 214–233.

Classen, C. C., Hughes, L., Clark, C., Hill Mohammed, B., Woods, P., & Beckett, B. (2021). A pilot RCT of a body-oriented group therapy for complex trauma survivors: An adaptation of sensorimotor psychotherapy. *Journal of Trauma & Dissociation*, *22*(1), 52–68.

Cloitre, M., Koenen, K. C., Cohen, L. R., & Han, H. (2002). Skills training in affective and interpersonal regulation followed by exposure: A phase-based treatment for PTSD related to childhood abuse. *Journal of Consulting and Clinical Psychology*, *70*(5), 1067.

Empson, S., Cuca, Y. P., Cocohoba, J., Dawson-Rose, C., Davis, K., & Machtinger, E. L. (2017). Seeking safety group therapy for co-occurring substance use disorder and PTSD among transgender women living with HIV: A pilot study. *Journal of Psychoactive Drugs, 49*(4), 344–351.

Gene-Cos, N., Fisher, J., Ogden, P., & Cantrell, A. (2016). Sensorimotor psychotherapy group therapy in the treatment of complex PTSD. *Annals of Psychiatry and Mental Health, 4*(6), 1080.

Giustino, T. F., Fitzgerald, P. J., & Maren, S. (2016). Revisiting propranolol and PTSD: Memory erasure or extinction enhancement? *Neurobiology of Learning and Memory, 130,* 26–33.

Grossman, P., & van Dam, N. T. (2011). Mindfulness, by any other name…: Trials and tribulations of sati in western psychology and science. *Contemporary Buddhism, 12*(1), 219–239.

Gudiño, O. G., Weis, J. R., Havens, J. F., Biggs, E. A., Diamond, U. N., Marr, M., … Cloitre, M. (2014). Group trauma-informed treatment for adolescent psychiatric inpatients: A preliminary uncontrolled trial. *Journal of Traumatic Stress, 27*(4), 496–500.

Healy, C. J., Lee, K. A., & D'Andrea, W. (2021). Using psychedelics with therapeutic intent is associated with lower shame and complex trauma symptoms in adults with histories of child maltreatment. *Chronic Stress, 5,* 1–12.

Jain, S., Ortigo, K., Gimeno, J., Baldor, D. A., Weiss, B. J., & Cloitre, M. (2020). A randomized controlled trial of brief skills training in affective and interpersonal regulation (STAIR) for veterans in primary care. *Journal of Traumatic Stress, 34*(4), 401–409.

Kuhfuß, M., Maldei, T., Hetmanek, A., & Baumann, N. (2021). Somatic experiencing–effectiveness and key factors of a body-oriented trauma therapy: A scoping literature review. *European Journal of Psychotraumatology, 12*(1), 1929023.

Lenz, A. S., Henesy, R., & Callender, K. (2016). Effectiveness of seeking safety for co-occurring posttraumatic stress disorder and substance use. *Journal of Counseling & Development, 94*(1), 51–61.

Linehan, M. M. (1987). Dialectical behavior therapy for borderline personality disorder: Theory and method. *Bulletin of the Menninger Clinic, 51*(3), 261.

Linehan, M. M. (2020). *Dialectical behavior therapy in clinical practice.* Guilford Publications.

Matsuno, E., & Israel, T. (2018). Psychological interventions promoting resilience among transgender individuals: Transgender resilience intervention model (TRIM). *The Counseling Psychologist, 46*(5), 632–655.

Mithoefer, M. C., Feduccia, A. A., Jerome, L., Mithoefer, A., Wagner, M., Walsh, Z., … Doblin, R. (2019). MDMA-assisted psychotherapy for treatment of PTSD: Study design and rationale for phase 3 trials based on pooled analysis of six phase 2 randomized controlled trials. *Psychopharmacology, 236*(9), 2735–2745.

Monteiro, N. M., & Wall, D. J. (2011). African dance as healing modality throughout the diaspora: The use of ritual and movement to work through trauma. *Journal of Pan African Studies, 4*(6), 234–252.

Najavits, L. (2002). *Seeking safety: A treatment manual for PTSD and substance abuse.* Guilford Publications.

Najavits, L. M., Weiss, R. D., Shaw, S. R., & Muenz, L. R. (1998). "Seeking safety": Outcome of a new cognitive-behavioral psychotherapy for women with posttraumatic stress disorder and substance dependence. *Journal of Traumatic Stress, 11*(3), 437–456.

Nguyen-Feng, V. N., Clark, C. J., & Butler, M. E. (2019). Yoga as an intervention for psychological symptoms following trauma: A systematic review and quantitative synthesis. *Psychological Services, 16*(3), 513.

Ogden, P. (2020). The different impact of trauma and relational stress on physiology, posture, and movement: Implications for treatment. *European Journal of Trauma & Dissociation,* 100172.

Payne, P., Levine, P. A., & Crane-Godreau, M. A. (2015). Somatic experiencing: Using interoception and proprioception as core elements of trauma therapy. *Frontiers in Psychology, 6*, 93.

Salihu, D., Wong, E. M., & Kwan, R. Y. (2021). Effects of an African circle dance programme on internally displaced persons with depressive symptoms: A quasi-experimental study. *International Journal of Environmental Research and Public Health, 18*(2), 843.

Sloan, C. A., Berke, D. S., & Shipherd, J. C. (2017). Utilizing a dialectical framework to inform conceptualization and treatment of clinical distress in transgender individuals. *Professional Psychology: Research and Practice, 48*(5), 301.

Smith, G., Morgans, A., Taylor, D. M., & Cameron, P. (2012). Use of the human dive reflex for the management of supraventricular tachycardia: A review of the literature. *Emergency Medicine Journal, 29*(8), 611–616.

Takahashi, L. M., Tobin, K., Li, F. Y., Proff, A., & Candelario, J. (2021). Healing transgender women of color in Los Angeles: A transgender-centric delivery of seeking safety. *International Journal of Transgender Health*, 1–16.

Tibbitts, D. C., Aicher, S. A., Sugg, J., Handloser, K., Eisman, L., Booth, L. D., & Bradley, R. D. (2021). Program evaluation of trauma-informed yoga for vulnerable populations. *Evaluation and Program Planning, 88*, 101946.

CHAPTER 11

PHASE 2: REPROCESSING

The reprocessing phase of treating trauma and stress is what many clinicians first think of when they think about trauma treatment. There are a number of different philosophies about what works and why in the reprocessing phase of trauma treatment. This chapter starts with an overview of the exposure-based treatments for PTSD specifically, then branches out to talk more eclectically about reprocessing-focused forms of intervention in an array of styles. It then discusses reprocessing and the intrapersonal phase of gender development, and ends with illustrations from the case histories.

THE EMOTION PROCESSING THEORY OF PTSD

There are several possible models for understanding PTSD and the various related symptoms. A popular model is emotion processing theory (EPT), which was first presented by Foa and Kozak (1986), and is the theoretical underpinning of prolonged exposure (PE) for PTSD as well as another exposure-based treatment, cognitive processing therapy (CPT). EPT is built on models of fear conditioning (Foa et al., 1989) and argues that exposure to a traumatic stressor creates an unprocessed activation of fear networks. This unprocessed activation of fear networks, EPT suggests, produces the symptoms of PTSD. Thus, the symptoms can be modified or eliminated by intentionally activating the fear network and restructuring that fear network while it is activated (Foa & Kozak, 1986). The treatments for PTSD that are based on EPT include an element of intentional imaginal exposure to the traumatic stressor in a controlled therapeutic context. A recent evaluation of the mechanisms of change associated with symptom reduction in PE discusses fear activation, within-session habituation, and between-session habituation as primary mechanisms (Brown et al., 2019). The activation and habituation cycles contribute to extinction of response to the feared stimulus.

While therapies focused on exposure and fear extinction have been around since the 1950s, prolonged exposure is likely the best known of the treatments stemming from EPT, and in some settings, PE is considered the gold standard of trauma treatment. The typical protocol is that, starting from the first (or sometimes second) session, the client describes the index trauma with as much sensory detail as possible, as if it were happening now. This imaginal exposure will typically take place two to three times per session. Subjective units of distress (SUDs) are monitored every five minutes, and the client is asked to stay in the memory until their SUDs decrease by about half. If the SUDs start low, the client is asked to describe the event in more vivid detail until the fear network is activated. The client is also audio-recorded. Homework generally consists of listening to the audio recording and also in vivo exposure to situations that the client avoids from fear. (For instance, if a client was assaulted in a parking lot at night, and therefore they avoid parking lots altogether, initial homework might be to spend five minutes in a parking lot during the day.) There are some variations in the timing and application, and there are a variety of clinicians' manuals and client workbooks available if you'd like to learn more. There was also a Dateline segment about PE if you'd like to hear more about it from the originator and see it in action. More recently, virtual reality exposure (VRE), which follows a similar treatment trajectory

DOI: 10.4324/9781003140740-12

as PE, but can intensify the imaginal exposure through the use of virtual reality, has been developed and tested alongside traditional PE. There do not appear to be robust differences in outcomes between PE and VRE, but a study of cisgender military personnel indicates that identity-based differences may have an impact on efficacy (Norr et al., 2018). This study found that younger soldiers with more hyperarousal symptoms tended to show greater responsivity to VRE. Sex assigned at birth was not considered in the final model, as the vast majority of the participants were AMAB. Studies that include heart rate and heart rate reactivity as outcome measures have found that PE and VRE reduced resting heart rate and heart rate reactivity in soldiers with PTSD (e.g., Bourassa et al., 2020).

Another reprocessing-focused treatment that is also based on EPT is CPT, which was originally designed for cisgender women who had been sexually assaulted. CPT uses writing for imaginal exposure rather than verbal retelling (see, e.g., Resick & Schnicke, 1992). Like PE, CPT is widely used in the VA system. It has also been adapted cross-culturally for no- and low-literacy users (see, e.g., Kaysen et al., 2013) and there is a mobile app for it.

In CPT, the client writes (or draws) the memory of the trauma and is encouraged in writing about the traumatic experience to integrate sensory detail and memories of thoughts and feelings at the time of exposure. Although CPT is based on EPT, it had a significantly smaller exposure component than PE and typically focuses more on restructuring beliefs and feelings related to the traumatic experience or at "stuck points" that may indicate conflict between previously held beliefs and the new information of the traumatic experience. A course of CPT is typically 12 weeks, and it can be offered in a group format. A study of cisgender adults comparing solely the written exposure component of CPT with a full course of CPT, however, found that the two were equitable for reducing symptoms of PTSD (Sloan et al., 2018). A study of clinician fidelity to the CPT model, as well as a disambiguation of relevant skills, indicates that clinicians achieve high levels of fidelity and are most successful when they are skilled in Socratic questioning and focus on assimilation (Farmer et al., 2017). For a review of PE, CPT, and trauma-focused cognitive behavioral therapy, see Watkins et al. (2018).

Although methods that operate from the EPT of PTSD are considered the standard of care in trauma treatment, there are a number of critiques of these models that I believe should be carefully considered when selecting them for implementation. One of the greatest critiques is the dropout rate. Although it varies from study to study, upwards of 40% of participants leave studies of these modalities prematurely (e.g., Kehle-Forbes et al., 2016). I'll also note that, as with all RCTs, prospective participants in these studies must already fit into a fairly narrow window of presentations in order to be included in the study symptoms. (Suicidality and psychotic-spectrum symptoms are common RCT rule outs, for instance, which means that the population included in the study is already very different than the population coming into the clinic.) I will qualify my next critique of PE because the research literature on it is not robust: it has been my experience that it can exacerbate existing symptoms or trigger the development of new symptoms. Anecdotally, I have seen a number of people in my practice who saw a previous clinician for PE and had the experience of getting worse. An opinion piece from the *New York Times* blog describes the experience of a veteran who had an adverse reaction to PE, although went on to benefit from CPT (Morris, 2015). Yet another critique is that identity matters in the selection of treatment, as does gender-based ideology. From what I have been able to discern, both PE and CPT were originally piloted in studies of cisgender women who had been sexually assaulted. They are now more likely to be used in a VA clinic than in other settings. I would argue that this directly relates to our ideas about the "toughness" of military personnel (including survivors of military sexual assault) versus civilian sexual assault survivors. There seems to be an ethos of "toughing it out" among PE devotees that lends itself well to a military environment. Again, it is difficult to draw direct, data-driven conclusions about the stereotypes relative to a TGD population because these treatment protocols do not have literature related to their use in explicitly TGD populations. Many of the studies related to these modalities have taken place in the Veterans Healthcare Administration, so we can assume that they include some TGD individuals, but the data regarding gender diversity have not been solicited or disambiguated in a meaningful way.

Of the TGD-specific literature that exists regarding exposure-based models, a recent study of trans-affirming narrative exposure therapy (TA-NET) provides a conceptual overview and case examples (Lange, 2020). There is also a helpful overview of evidence-based practices for PTSD as pertains to the broader LGBTQ community, which discusses PE and CPT, as well as treatments geared toward emotion regulation (such as the unified protocol) with tailoring for sexual minority communities (namely a protocol called ESTEEM or effective skills to empower effective men), but this review notes that most treatments that have been tailored to LGBTQ communities focus on (mostly cisgender) men who have sex with (mostly cisgender) men (Livingston et al., 2020). This review also notes that evidence-based treatments, such as CPT and PE, were designed to treat PTSD emerging from strictly defined Criterion A stressors. This is, in my opinion, another critique of the exposure-based modalities, although others may see this as a strength.

OTHER WAYS OF ADDRESSING TRAUMA AND STRESS

In my own practice, it is fairly uncommon for me to use EPT-based protocols as front-line treatments in work with TGD people who have been exposed to trauma and stress. As mentioned above, a portion of my clients have already received some form of exposure therapy. This could mean that those people have already had their PTSD successfully treated, and they come to me looking to work on other posttraumatic sequelae. It could also mean that these modalities are less successful with a TGD population, or marginalized populations that experience a blend of Criterion A stressors and minority stressors, than they are in RCTs. It could also mean that the people who specifically seek out different kinds of treatment are the people who have had no benefit from, or adverse reactions to, those styles of treatment. But, realistically, the question of whether a strict exposure model is necessary or desirable for treating trauma is a topic of significant debate in the field of trauma therapy (see Dimaggio, 2019, for a thoughtful overview). Probably, the answer is that we don't know for sure—that it depends on the client and on the clinician.

Some reprocessing-based model for PTSD, CPTSD, and additional symptoms related to trauma and stress are not strictly exposure-based or not built on the model of EPT. One, eye-movement desensitization and reprocessing (EMDR), has a significant exposure component, although it is based on what the developer describes as the adaptive information processing model (see Shapiro & Laliotis, 2011). This model postulates that the traumatic memories are incompletely processed and thus are encoded in memory in an inalterable form that carries too much sensory information. Thus, the focus of EMDR is on accessing those incompletely processed memories and updating them with new information and insights. EMDR focuses on remembered images as opposed to verbal retelling of the traumatic memory. The client is asked to imagine a particular scene from the traumatic memory in great detail while being cued to move their eyes from side to side (or sometimes engage in another form of bilateral engagement). One theory behind the posited efficacy of the eye movements is that they activate the brain bilaterally, aiding in the transfer of the traumatic memory from the right hemisphere to the left. Thus, memories that have been stored in non-verbal memory can be consolidated and restructured verbally (for a review of studies related to EMDR, including analysis of the function of the eye movements, see Landin-Romero, 2018).

Interpersonal therapy (IPT) is an example of a model that has components of reprocessing, but is not focused on exposure. IPT was originally developed for treating depression, but has also been manualized for the treatment of PTSD (see Bleiberg & Markowitz, 2019). IPT for PTSD explicitly utilizes the medical model for defining PTSD, in that it identifies the client as sick, while reassuring the client that they are sick because something bad happened to them, and that this is not their fault. It then focuses on here-and-now interventions for identifying affect, and working through interpersonal difficulties. While the client is not encouraged to revisit the trauma, they are asked to tolerate uncomfortable emotions related to the experience of the trauma. The clinician normalizes these feelings and encourages the client to find new avenues for interpersonal relatedness. In terms of efficacy, one study compared IPT for PTSD with both PE and relaxation therapy for PTSD in a group of cisgender individuals (Markowitz et al., 2015). There were no statistically significant differences in effect between the treatment conditions, but IPT did have a lower dropout rate than the comparison conditions and also proved more effective for individuals reporting sexual trauma. For a meta-analysis of IPT for PTSD, see Althobaiti et al. (2020).

In terms of IPT for use in TGD populations, there are case studies of clinicians using IPT to help with "role transition" as adults are in the transition process (Barbisan et al., 2020; Budge, 2013). One provides four examples of the ways in which the core elements of IPT can be used for addressing role transition: evaluating the old role, encouraging the expression of affect related to transition, building a new set of social skills, and establishing social supports (Budge). This author also speaks to the importance of holding hope for clients in the midst of a sometimes-difficult period of life. The other case study contributes themes of mourning the loss of the old role, celebrating the positive aspects of the new role, and acquiring new role-related skills (Barbisan). While these may translate into useful interventions for trauma and stress-related symptoms in TGD people with PTSD, there is not enough literature to evaluate this specifically.

Internal Family Systems (IFS) is also not explicitly reprocessing-based, but does incorporate elements of reprocessing in attempts to understand and welcome various parts of ourselves that may have been pushed aside or blocked from our conscious awareness. IFS suggests that some internal subdivision of the mind is not only non-pathological, but a necessary and healthy part of life (see Schwartz, 2013). According to the IFS model, there is a core Self, and this Self is protected by parts labeled Managers, Firefighters, and Exiles. Exiles hold the traumatic and painful pieces of our experience that might swamp or psychologically destroy us, while other protector parts either defend against the awareness of the Exile or attempt to soothe this part when it has become activated. While there is less research literature related to IFS, it can have value for people who have experienced trauma and stress as a way of normalizing the experience of a fracture sense of self, or a divided self-state. It also offers a name for those parts of ourselves that hold traumatic memory. This can allow the opportunity to integrate the traumatic material as something that absolutely impacted the person, while recognizing that they have a whole and healthy core Self that has been protected by many of the choices and behaviors they may not like about themselves. I mention IFS here as several TGD individuals I know have found it to be helpful, but I myself am not very conversant with the model.

PSYCHODYNAMIC MODELS

While I am influenced by all of these modalities and more in my reprocessing work with TGD people, I am most influenced by psychodynamic and interpersonal theories. Frankly, there is not a lot of data at the RCT level to indicate if these are helpful for the sequelae of trauma and stress at all, let alone with TGD people. I think that this is for a number of different reasons. One is that ongoing therapy is just that—ongoing. It is not designed for a 12- to 16-week manualized treatment, and it is difficult to assess what constitutes fidelity to the model. This makes it harder to study through an RCT; it also means that it will be difficult to obtain grant funding to study it, that many agencies can't afford to offer it, and that many people who want it and could benefit from it can't access it. So, there are these tremendous elements of time, money, and insurance coverage, all of which are significant barriers to access of treatment of any kind and get larger with ongoing treatment.

I think there's another barrier to psychodynamic models of treatment, however, which is the anxiety of the clinician. Treating trauma is hard and sometimes painful work. Treating trauma can cause a clinician to be more fearful about the world, to worry that the world is out of control. To put it bluntly, the world *is* out of control, and no-one is fully protected from the horrible things that humans do to one another. It can feel especially reassuring, in this context, to feel as if we have a way of knowing that we're doing everything "right." Manualized treatments with a lot of RCT data can offer this reassurance—we're doing the treatment "right" if we achieve fidelity to the model, and if this means a high dropout rate, well, that's a client issue, not a clinician issue. I see this as a corollary to clinicians who, in work with TGD individuals, get so preoccupied by trying to make absolutely sure the client will never regret transition that they create obstacles and barriers to medical transition.

There is yet another issue with using psychodynamic models of care for the reprocessing phase of trauma work with specifically TGD people: many psychodynamic theories are rooted in pathologizing notions of gender and ideas about the desirability of gendered "normativity." If psychodynamic models play a role in your work, I'd encourage you to read psychodynamic theory being generated by and for TGD people as well as theory generated by and for people who hold other marginalized identities. For TGD-centered theoretical perspectives you might see Saketopoulou (2020), Hansbury (2017), or Pula (2015) as starting points, or if you prefer case histories you might see Chang and Singh (2016) or McConnell (2018). For an overview of the development of psychodynamic theory for the treatment of PTSD and CPTSD, see Spermon et al. (2010).

Reduced to the simplest form, psychodynamic philosophy assumes that we have drives, motivations, and defenses of which we are only partially aware, often rooted in childhood experiences, but there are any number of elaborations on this that have developed over the years.

One recent article about the psychodynamic treatment of trauma takes the interesting approach of comparing three cases of cisgender Belgian survivors of childhood maltreatment, identifying consistent themes across the cases (van Nieuwenhove & Meganck, 2020). These authors articulate a shared core desire among the clients—the desire to not be hurt—which results in an interpersonal difficulty with doing things that might be upsetting to others. Others are perceived as rejecting, angry, or untrustworthy, and thus the only way to meet the core need of being loved and accepted is to comply, which elicits anger and resentment in the individual complying. I find this to be broadly applicable in my own work. You read about some of the ways I endeavor to help a client feel safe in their bodies in the previous chapter. Some of the ways in which I endeavor to encourage them to feel safe with me include consistency and regularity (starting on time and ending on time, being conscientious about doing things I say I am going to do and taking accountability when I forget or get it wrong), and working to build awareness of counter-transference reactions I might have that could elicit a desire to lash out or withhold. This means taking my own development and self-care seriously. I also work to build a safe relationship with clients by talking openly about my identities. Frankly, I'd greatly prefer to be a blank slate onto which clients could freely project, as this is a much safer and more comfortable position for me. It is a position of disavowed subjectivity, however, and I believe this decreases safety in the therapy space.

Another way in which I endeavor to approach reprocessing is that I commit to believing whatever my clients tell me about their traumatic experiences. People who have experienced trauma and stress have often been disbelieved or had their experiences minimized (or both). Because of this, and because of physiological dysregulation, dissociation, alexithymia, etc., people who have experienced trauma can sound like they are lying, especially when they talk about trauma. I do not believe it is my job to try to sniff out the literal truth of what happened. I do believe that it's my responsibility to profoundly believe in the symbolic truth of what my client is saying and not get too married to literal "truth." So, I try start from a baseline of unwavering belief. This means engaging with the content that the client presents on its own terms and stopping myself when I want to ask a lot of questions about internal inconsistencies.

Second, I listen for repetition and gaps. When children are traumatized, we look for repetitive play to guide our interventions and questions. With adults, words and themes are frequently the equivalent of play. In dynamic work, someone telling the same story over and over again in a rigid and inflexible way indicates a block. Listening for a word said with atypical fervor or repeated frequently, and simply repeating the word back to the person with a questioning intonation can open the door for a new direction in the story. When language becomes vague, on the other hand, it may be that the person literally can't access those details or doesn't feel safe providing them. A clinician can nod to this gap by saying, "wait, I'm confused—make the link between A and B for me." Or, if the problem seems to be lack of safety for accessing those details, a clinician can consider an intervention along the lines of, "let's slow down for a moment—how is your body doing with this conversation?"

In addition to addressing the content around repetition and gaps, you may choose to comment on body language at these moments. When people are talking around a trauma, they often lean forward or back, avert their eyes, flush, blanche, grip their stomachs, or hug themselves. Their voice might get high and fast or low and slow. They may grip their chair or even stand up and begin pacing. They might seem uninterruptable or we might struggle to redirect their attention. This might not tell us exactly what is going on, but it indicates something big is going on. In these moments, I believe, our responsibility is to manage the pacing and our own reactions so that there is room for the client to say what they need to say, while still experiencing us as active in the treatment and connected to their process.

Listening for repetition and gaps, and noting body language, can be quite subtle. Then there are times when a frozen or explosive reaction to a trauma trigger is not at all subtle. For instance, when people have had a great need to tell their story frequently, but not necessarily in a therapeutic context, they often report it in a flat, affectless "script" that they struggle to deviate from. This can happen with children who are involved in the foster care system, for instance, and may have had to repeat their stories of maltreatment many times to DFCS workers or members of the court for the purposes of documentation. I also see this frequently with adults who have been involved in the court system, who had to find a way to tell their stories on the stand without breaking down, or refugees who have had to internalize coaching from lawyers and advocates regarding the most effective way of communicating about the abuse they have suffered. In short, any time a person has had to repeat their trauma narrative for the purposes of a system, rather than for their own benefit and healing, it runs the risk of becoming a script that the person can read off of, but not really deviate from. Sometimes these people can look as if their trauma has been metabolized, as they can report truly horrific experiences without turning a hair. We might have to hear it from them two or three times before we realize that every word, every pause, is predetermined, and there is no flexibility in the reporting. The story, then, gets reified and rigid, and it gets harder for the person to grow in relationship to the experience. It starts to feel static and frozen, and this can also be difficult for a clinician to work with. In general, I find it easiest to simply note what I observe. "I can see you have told this story a number of times. It sounds like it's a bit stuck or frozen. Does it feel that way?" The most common reply that I get with this question is, "yes, but it's the only way I can tell my story." At which point I can remind my client (or tell them if I never have) that we are not in a rush, and suggest it might feel better to tell me the narrative of their trauma when we connect with it in a different way. Just to reiterate on the timing front, if you *are* in a situation where you don't have adequate time in which to not rush (you are operating within an agency's session limits, for instance) I would recommend sticking with safety-focused forms of treatment. Rushing through reprocessing is like trying to rush through re-roofing when a storm is brewing—better to shore things up and come back to the project when there is more time.

When a piece of content feels less like it's frozen and more like it's explosive, this presents a different set of challenges. People who have experienced trauma may find that they form relationships very quickly, and, as mentioned in previous chapters, that these relationships burn hot and fast. This can have the effect, in therapy, of the client wanting to tell all of the traumatic events all at once, and it might come pouring out in a seemingly-unstoppable flow. This can be very dysregulating for the client and clinician alike, and also runs the risk of feeding into a pattern of idealization (my therapist will fix me!) followed by disappointment and devaluation (my therapist is a useless quack). It can also happen that people feel pressured to tell a clinician everything all at once because they think it will speed up the process, or that the therapist won't "get it" until they client has told everything. I find the intervention for the rapid flow is the same as above—deliberately slowing everything down. I tend to say something along the lines of

> I definitely want to hear everything you have to say, and I think I can be most helpful to you if we know each other a little more before moving into trauma work. I don't yet know what comes up for you when you feel overwhelmed, or the kinds of things that are helpful to you when you *do* feel overwhelmed, and I'd hate to encourage you to share in a way that feels like too much.

Before you try it, if you decide to and you haven't already, I'll just mention that slowing down a trauma disclosure is very uncomfortable. But it is quite rewarding, in that as the story begins to shift and there is a bit more lightness and freedom. The relief in the room can be palpable. This intervention also allows more opportunity for the pattern-recognition and interpretation that typify psychodynamic psychotherapy.

HOW DOES THIS FIT WITH THE PROCESS
OF GENDER DEVELOPMENT?

There are some similarities in the reprocessing phase of therapy and the meso-level or combined person and social processes of gender development described in Chapter 8, although
this does not mean that they necessarily happen in parallel in the context of therapy. In the
safety and stabilization phase, as with the micro-level of gender development, the focus is on
the individual's experience of their body, including finding ways to feel safe in the body as it
is, and reflecting on what might help the body move through the world in a less burdened,
more authentic way. In this meso-level of gender development, the focus is on relationships
with important people, potentially including the therapist, and seeing one's gender reflected
and affirmed by those important others. The reprocessing phase, as I understand it, is also
deeply rooted in relational processes. When a client begins to feel safer in their relationship,
they may begin to test the safety parameters of the therapeutic relationship, and this may
take the form of gender disclosures, trauma disclosures, or disclosures that contain elements
of both trauma and gender. Being witnessed in our experiences of ourselves is powerful.

REPROCESSING AND THE CASE HISTORIES

Reprocessing with Advika largely focused on disclosures of gendered trauma as it unfolded
in the context of her particular family and cultural context. As Advika became more able
to feel their body, it became increasingly evident to both of us that they very much wanted
to begin using estrogen. She described great fear that her parents would disown her if she
did decide to use estrogen, and one day, rather laughingly, told me that they had already
threatened to do so. Because Advika said this so lightly, sandwiched in between two equally
lighthearted statements, I almost didn't catch it. They did give a rather sideways, invitational
glance when they said it that I *did* notice, though, so I asked to back up a step and asked
what they had meant. Advika talked about a memory from childhood of seeing a group of
hijra show up at a wedding. (Hijra are members of a third gender in India and often present at religious ceremonies. They are generally disrespected and frequently make a living
from begging and sex work. Many are abandoned by their families of origin in childhood.
Academic resources that were helpful to me regarding cultural context for work with Advika
were articles about the oppression of Indian gender and sexual minorities, particularly as
advanced by British colonialism, such as Hinchy (2017) and Loh (2018). I also consulted
popular media. While these things were helpful to me, my understanding is limited, and of
course not guided by lived experience.) Advika reported that her mother had hissed at her,
"See? This is what we are saving you from." Advika did not understand the reference very
well at the time, but later remembered that this was shortly after their nanny had been fired,
and their grandmother had taken over the role of primary caregiver. Once these pieces fell
together for her, she became more and more secretive about her cache of "girl clothes,"
and this coincided with a growing sense of disconnection from her body. They noticed that
refraining from eating helped fuel this disconnection and the sense that their body and their
brain were two separate entities. But a growing sense of safety in her body had led to her
noticing desires for things like food, sleep, sex, longer hair, softer skin, and breasts. These
desires had brought the long-suppressed fear, shame, grief, and anger about early childhood
mis-attunement to the surface as well as fear about a possible loss of family. The reprocessing of familial mis-attunement was influenced by my American sense of the role of family,

and Advika's worries about how that sense might impact our reprocessing related to TGD people and familial connection. Advika was willing to describe the expectations placed on an only child (considered an only son) in the context of a family structure that had much more interdependence than white American families with no immigrant family members of a comparable class background. And in all honesty, if I had observed this degree of connection in the family of a wealthy, white, non-immigrant, TGD person, I may have inquired further into the health of the system. For instance, Advika would have been unable to initiate estrogen without their family's awareness because they and their parents contributed to a single bank account and their father paid the bills, which I would consider enmeshed if taking place in white American family. Until I exhibited some understanding of this familial interdependence and clearly indicated that I did not find it pathological, it was dangerous for Advika to critique her family to me. Even then, they were very cautious about doing so and very protective of the family unit. So while, even in retrospect, Advika's ready eagerness to forgive her parents and think the absolute best of them seems somewhat defensive to me, I also believe her eagerness to fold more seamlessly back into the family system was culturally specific. I also believe that interpreting it with more skepticism or probing would have been (rightly) injurious to their trust in our relationship. This was really important for us to talk about openly because, for Advika, reprocessing the familial mis-attunement was much more difficult and more central than reprocessing the Criterion A stressor they had experienced, and also directly related to the meso level of gender development. She was not going to be able to move forward in expressing her authentic gender without the approval—or at least the non-disapproval—of her parents. To get that, they were going to have to come to terms with their gender to the point of being able to tolerate their parents' reactions to their disclosure of gender identity, and help their parents through the process, whatever it might be. I would say that Advika experienced significant rupture, and we had to figure out a way to reprocess it without knowing if she was going to experience a replication of that, and also without being too explicit in naming it. The most helpful technique I had available to me during this process was a psychodynamic stance of not siding with one part of the conflict. If, when she talked and talked about how great her parents were, I had pointed to the rupture, she would have doubled down on their greatness. If, when they edged toward talking about their feelings of hurt and betrayal, I had redirected toward parental greatness, they would have felt guilty and silenced. A more neutral—although still affirming and open—stance was necessary.

With Daniel reprocessing was quite different. Daniel was very in touch with his dysphoria, his desires for his body, and his gender expression, and this did not change at all as he started feeling safer in his body and less anxious in therapy. What did start to shift was his relationship with alcohol. Instead of drinking moderately most nights, he began cycling. He would drink lightly for a night or two, then maybe very heavily one night, then abstain entirely for a night or two, in a shifting pattern. He was drinking less overall, and his periods of abstinence helped him feel confident that he would be able to go without alcohol entirely in the days leading up to surgery and while he was on pain killers afterward, but he remained unhappy with his pattern of alcohol consumption and worried about the effect on his health.

After tracking this with him for a while, I gently asked him if he thought there was anything happening on those nights he did choose to drink heavily that might be contributing to that choice. He quickly replied "No" and abruptly looked away. I decided it was a premature question and left it there.

Over our next few sessions, Daniel experienced a flight to health. He talked about his new job, his workout regimen, the weather, and what he was watching on television that he thought I'd really enjoy. Clinically speaking, it was pretty boring. He would occasionally seem to be leading toward something important, and then very smoothly switch conversation in mid-stream. This conversational change in direction coincided with physical indications of discomfort—a slight tapping of his finger, or his eyes would dart to the clock over my shoulder as if he couldn't wait to get out of there. "You feeling anxious?" I'd ask. "I'm ok," he'd reply tersely.

And then one day he came into the office in visible distress. In this particular instance, though, what he needed to communicate was kind of pouring out of him, and because I had never seen him pour out distressing content before, I didn't slow him down in the way I might have with another client. This was an error in clinical judgment. The trauma that was coming up for him was from the first time he had sex, and he related his episodes of heavy drinking to triggers that reminded him of that experience. I want to be very clear that I identify his experience as sexual assault. For him it felt more complicated, as he had (and has) strong feelings of attachment, affinity, and regard for his assailant, who was also his boyfriend and superior officer.

As I mentioned, I made the mistake of not interjecting when he told this story the first couple of times he told it. He would tell me in a fixed and rigid format about how the two of them had been experimenting with sexual activity in the preceding weeks, but that they were taking it slow, and then how they had too much to drink and "got carried away." Daniel described not being ready, having physical pain during penetration, being surprised and scared by the sudden violation of trust, and also his assailant's expression of hurt and anger at the "accusation" when Daniel tried to talk about his experience with him later. This left Daniel feeling confused, wondering if he was making a big deal out of nothing, and with nowhere to take his complicated feelings. His sexual relationship with this person continued, and he described a feeling of splitting when he had sex, noticing that his body was feeling hyperaroused (as well as, sometimes, sexually aroused) while his mind was distant or even absent. As an adult, he mostly drank heavily when he was sexually active, or overwhelmed by memories of sexual maltreatment.

After Daniel repeated this memory to me in the same, rote fashion a couple of times, without experiencing relief or change, I noticed that I was feeling disconnected from his story in a way that is pretty uncommon for me. This internal clinical information, coupled with his formulaic repetition, led me to feel I should experiment with slowing him down. When relating this story, he would sit with his face turned aside so that I was looking at him almost in profile. The next time he came in and turned his head that way I intervened before he started talking. "Hey, I think the memory of what happened to you when you were a kid is strong today, is that right?" He turned more toward me and looked surprised, which made sense because I rarely tell someone where we are starting. He agreed, saying it had been on his mind and he wanted to talk more about it. I asked if we could try talking about it in a different way, and he wanted more details before he agreed. I told him what I'd noticed about him turning away, and asked if we could use the times he wanted to turn away as a sign to slow down, and he was willing to experiment with that. I also asked if he would be willing to keep an eye on his heart rate and we would stop and do a breathing exercise or try something different if it got over 100 bpm and he agreed to that. We did not make it very far into the retelling that day, we spent a lot of time on breathing exercises. The next time we met, we made it further, and a new detail emerged. His assailant had said something that had made it clear that he knew Daniel was saying "no" in the moment, and that he was going to continue anyway. Daniel repeated it to me as if he were the assailant, with a kind of careless disregard for pain, and then quickly turned his face away. "You felt ashamed," I said. "Still do," he said with a short, dry laugh. The next time we talked about this experience, there was more freedom and flexibility in how he related the story, and his shame levels and reported alcohol use started to decline.

Shai used trauma disclosure sadomasochistically. They would ratchet up the intensity of what they were disclosing while smirking or glaring at me. The first few times I interjected to slow things down, they would sneer and say, "Oh, I had to live through that and you can't even handle hearing about it?" They sometimes used non-suicidal self-injury in the same way, either rolling up their sleeves in an exaggerated fashion to show new cuts and burns, or picking up small items in my office and pressing them against their skin while clearly gauging my reaction. I fell into an enactment around this with Shai, and for a while I was withholding in my reaction, acting impervious to these behaviors while internally angry and irritated. Fortunately for both me and Shai, I have trauma-informed colleagues with whom I regularly consult, and I had the opportunity to talk with these colleagues about my difficulties in this relationship. They encouraged me to take the risk of being more open about my internal process with this person, and talking with them also made my own internal processes feel less fraught (and thus something that could be therapeutically shared). I was also reading some excellent fat justice theory at the time, which helped me think about the ways in which internalized anti-fat bias might be leading me to see Shai as more aggressive and (psychologically) older than they were. Finally, I was in the process of learning more about autism, and was able to recognize the possibility that I was interpreting some elements of their communication as aggressive instead of being open to the possibility that those elements were a function of my centering allistic styles of communication as normative. I wasn't sure about any of this, but thinking through these possibilities, and the wholehearted support and gentle pushing of people I had the chance to consult with, gave me the opportunity to experiment with something different instead of stewing in my irritation or deciding I just couldn't work with Shai.

The next time Shai sneered at me, I said something along the lines of, "you know, it kind of seems like you're trying to get a rise out of me." Thanks to my consultation, I was able to share this in way that was interested and friendly, but not accusatory or overinvested in any particular response from them. "Wow, you're a regular Dr. Fraud," they replied.

"Why do you want me to be angry at you? What purpose does it serve for you?" Again, I was very aware of trying to remain curious and nonjudgmental asking this question.

"Entertainment, mostly. But also so I know how you react when you're angry. Shows me how you're going to try to hurt me."

I couldn't pretend this answer didn't break my heart a little, and I'm sure that was visible on my face and in my voice when I said, "I see. Well, actually, let me make sure I understand. When people are angry at you, they lash out at you. You want to see what it's like when I lash out. Is that right?"

"I guess," they shrugged.

"OK. Well you should know that it doesn't make me feel angry when you talk about the things that happened to you, or at least I don't feel angry at you. I feel sad that those things happened to you, and sometimes I feel angry at the people who did those things to you, but I don't feel angry at you."

"You don't seem sad," they said, in a very small and quiet voice.

"That's my mistake, and I'm sorry. I will definitely let you know when I feel sad about the things you're telling me as we move forward. OK?"

"OK."

"But I do feel angry when you scratch at yourself with (one of the items on my office end table), so please don't do that anymore. OK?"

"I'll think about it."

Although this didn't emerge in the preceding conversation *per se*, Shai also had a lot of nuance and complexity around gender development. I ultimately realized that they had very prickly responses around the things they desperately wanted me to ask about, so when they had a prickly response I'd suggest we do some safety techniques before I asked again. Their defensive maneuvering was to go swiftly and immediately on the offense, and I respected this as a strategy while at the same time hoping to engender some greater strategic flexibility for my own sake as well as theirs. I felt that there was a shift on multiple fronts when they showed more willingness to talk about their gender identity and their frustrations with people who assumed they aligned with their birth-assigned sex, and also with (often other TGD) people who assumed they were partway into a binary transition.

IN SUM

I hope this offers an overview of various ways to theorize about, formulate, and engage in the process of reprocessing. I come to the end of this chapter feeling that there is so much more to say, but also excited and eager to jump into the role of community in the treatment of trauma. Ready? Here we go.

WORKS CITED

Althobaiti, S., Kazantzis, N., Ofori-Asenso, R., Romero, L., Fisher, J., Mills, K. E., & Liew, D. (2020). Efficacy of interpersonal psychotherapy for post-traumatic stress disorder: A systematic review and meta-analysis. *Journal of Affective Disorders, 264*, 286–294.

Barbisan, G. K., Moura, D. H., Lobato, M. I. R., & Da Rocha, N. S. (2020). Interpersonal psychotherapy for gender dysphoria in a transgender woman. *Archives of Sexual Behavior, 49*(2), 787–791.

Bourassa, K. J., Stevens, E. S., Katz, A. C., Rothbaum, B. O., Reger, G. M., & Norr, A. M. (2020). The impact of exposure therapy on resting heart rate and heart rate reactivity among active-duty soldiers with posttraumatic stress disorder. *Psychosomatic Medicine, 82*(1), 108–114.

Bleiberg, K. L., & Markowitz, J. C. (2019). Interpersonal psychotherapy for PTSD: Treating trauma without exposure. *Journal of Psychotherapy Integration, 29*(1), 15.

Brown, L. A., Zandberg, L. J., & Foa, E. B. (2019). Mechanisms of change in prolonged exposure therapy for PTSD: Implications for clinical practice. *Journal of Psychotherapy Integration, 29*(1), 6.

Budge, S. L. (2013). Interpersonal psychotherapy with transgender clients. *Psychotherapy, 50*(3), 356.

Chang, S. C., & Singh, A. A. (2016). Affirming psychological practice with transgender and gender nonconforming people of color. *Psychology of Sexual Orientation and Gender Diversity, 3*(2), 140–147. https://doi.org/10.1037/sgd0000153

Dimaggio, G. (2019). To expose or not to expose? The integrative therapist and posttraumatic stress disorder. *Journal of Psychotherapy Integration, 29*(1), 1.

Farmer, C. C., Mitchell, K. S., Parker-Guilbert, K., & Galovski, T. E. (2017). Fidelity to the cognitive processing therapy protocol: Evaluation of critical elements. *Behavior Therapy, 48*(2), 195–206.

Foa, E. B., & Kozak, M. J. (1986). Emotional processing of fear: Exposure to corrective information. *Psychological Bulletin, 99*(1), 20.

Foa, E. B., Steketee, G., & Rothbaum, B. O. (1989). Behavioral/cognitive conceptualizations of post-traumatic stress disorder. *Behavior Therapy, 20*(2), 155–176.

Hansbury, G. (2017). Unthinkable anxieties: Reading transphobic countertransferences in a century of psychoanalytic writing. *Transgender Studies Quarterly, 4*(3–4), 384–404.

Hinchy, J. (2017). The eunuch archive: Colonial records of non-normative gender and sexuality in India. *Culture, Theory and Critique, 58*(2), 127–146.

Kaysen, D., Lindgren, K., Zangana, G. A. S., Murray, L., Bass, J., & Bolton, P. (2013). Adaptation of cognitive processing therapy for treatment of torture victims: Experience in Kurdistan, Iraq. *Psychological Trauma: Theory, Research, Practice, and Policy, 5*(2), 184.

Kehle-Forbes, S. M., Meis, L. A., Spoont, M. R., & Polusny, M. A. (2016). Treatment initiation and dropout from prolonged exposure and cognitive processing therapy in a VA outpatient clinic. *Psychological Trauma: Theory, Research, Practice, and Policy, 8*(1), 107.

Landin-Romero, R., Moreno-Alcazar, A., Pagani, M., & Amann, B. L. (2018). How does eye movement desensitization and reprocessing therapy work? A systematic review on suggested mechanisms of action. *Frontiers in Psychology, 9*, 1395.

Lange, T. M. (2020). Trans-affirmative narrative exposure therapy (TA-NET): A therapeutic approach for targeting minority stress, internalized stigma, and trauma reactions among gender diverse adults. *Practice Innovations, 5*(3), 230–245. https://doi.org/10.1037/pri0000126

Livingston, N. A., Berke, D., Scholl, J., Ruben, M., & Shipherd, J. C. (2020). Addressing diversity in PTSD treatment: Clinical considerations and guidance for the treatment of PTSD in LGBTQ populations. *Current Treatment Options in Psychiatry, 7*(2), 53–69.

Loh, J. U. (2018). Transgender identity, sexual versus gender 'rights' and the tools of the Indian state. *Feminist Review, 119*(1), 39–55.

Markowitz, J. C., Petkova, E., Neria, Y., Van Meter, P. E., Zhao, Y., Hembree, E., … Marshall, R. D. (2015). Is exposure necessary? A randomized clinical trial of interpersonal psychotherapy for PTSD. *American Journal of Psychiatry, 172*(5), 430–440.

McConnell, E. A. (2018). Risking it anyway: An adolescent case study of trauma, sexual and gender identities, and relationality. *Issues in Mental Health Nursing, 39*(1), 73–82.

Morris, D. J. (2015, January 17). After PTSD, more trauma. *The New York Times*, Opinions. https://opinionator.blogs.nytimes.com/2015/01/17/after-ptsd-more-trauma/

Norr, A. M., Smolenski, D. J., Katz, A. C., Rizzo, A. A., Rothbaum, B. O., Difede, J., … Reger, G. M. (2018). Virtual reality exposure versus prolonged exposure for PTSD: Which treatment for whom? *Depression and Anxiety, 35*(6), 523–529.

Pula, J. (2015). Understanding gender through the lens of transgender experience. *Journal of Psychoanalytic Inquiry, Special Volume of Gender, 35*(8), 809–822.

Resick, P. A., & Schnicke, M. K. (1992). Cognitive processing therapy for sexual assault victims. *Journal of Consulting and Clinical Psychology, 60*(5), 748.

Saketopoulou, A. (2020). Thinking psychoanalytically, thinking better: Reflections on transgender. *The International Journal of Psychoanalysis, 101*(5), 1019–1030.

Schwartz, R. C. (2013). Moving from acceptance toward transformation with internal family systems therapy (IFS). *Journal of Clinical Psychology, 69*(8), 805–816.

Shapiro, F., & Laliotis, D. (2011). EMDR and the adaptive information processing model: Integrative treatment and case conceptualization. *Clinical Social Work Journal, 39*(2), 191–200.

Sloan, D. M., Marx, B. P., Lee, D. J., & Resick, P. A. (2018). A brief exposure-based treat-
    ment vs cognitive processing therapy for posttraumatic stress disorder: A randomized
    noninferiority clinical trial. *JAMA Psychiatry, 75*(3), 233–239.
Spermon, D., Darlington, Y., & Gibney, P. (2010). Psychodynamic psychotherapy for com-
    plex trauma: Targets, focus, applications, and outcomes. *Psychology Research and Behavior
    Management, 3*, 119.
van Nieuwenhove, K., & Meganck, R. (2020). Core interpersonal patterns in complex
    trauma and the process of change in psychodynamic therapy: A case comparison study.
    Frontiers in Psychology, 11, 122.
Watkins, L. E., Sprang, K. R., & Rothbaum, B. O. (2018). Treating PTSD: A review of evi-
    dence-based psychotherapy interventions. *Frontiers in Behavioral Neuroscience, 12*, 258.

CHAPTER 12

PHASE 3: FINDING AND BUILDING AFFIRMING COMMUNITIES

While there are a number of theories behind the belief that social connection is important for recovery and resilience in people who have been exposed to trauma and stress, I'll focus here on attachment theory, as this theory also has a few studies focused on TGD participants. Polyvagal theory might also be another interesting direction in which to reflect, but beyond the scope of this chapter (see Porges & Dana, 2018).

Attachment theory was initially developed by John Bowlby (1973) and operationalized through the work of Mary Ainsworth (1978; for an early cross-cultural meta-analysis, see Van Ijzendoorn & Kroonenberg, 1988). Attachment theory helps us understand the relationship between children and their primary caregivers (originally formulated as the mom who had birthed the child, in the context of a white nuclear family) and has been extended to the investigation of relationships between adults and children in different kinds of family constellations and also to better understand adults in romantic relationships. Most recently, the book *Polysecure: Attachment, Trauma, and Consensual Nonmonogamy* outlines attachment theory as relates to all kinds of romantic and sexual relationships between consenting adults, although centered on cisgender experiences (Fern, 2020). Attachment styles were originally formulated as secure, anxious, avoidant, and disorganized, with disorganized attachment predicted by trauma and stress in the home (Main & Solomon, 1986). Different attachment styles seem to be associated with different levels of oxytocin, the hormone and neuropeptide associated with love and affiliation (among many other things; for an overview of the role of oxytocin and the impact of trauma and ACEs on the production of oxytocin, see Sharma et al., 2020).

Attachment theory has been explored in Australian TGD youth (Kozlowska et al., 2021) and Italian TGD adults (Giovanardi et al., 2018): please note that these studies conceptualize gender and TGD identities differently than I do). It has also been studied in American women (Sizemore et al., 2021). The youth study indicated that, while TGD youth presenting to a gender clinic were at greater risk of attachment disruption than a group of cisgender controls, their attachment patterns were not significantly different than a group of cisgender controls with psychiatric diagnoses. Attachment disruption in the TGD group was predicted by family structure and by exposure to ACEs. The study of adult women found that secure attachment moderated the risk of depression and substance use in survivors of childhood sexual abuse. I have not seen studies specific to oxytocin and attachment in TGD people, but I believe this would be an interesting area for future research, as estrogen increases oxytocin binding, and thus HRT could potentially help create conditions for fascinating within-participant longitudinal research.

Whatever the theoretical rationale, integration or reintegration into the community is an important component in the lives of people experiencing the sequelae of exposure to traumatic and stressful experiences. Social support buffers people who have experienced Criterion A stressors against developing PTSD or mitigates the severity of the symptoms (for a meta-analysis, see Zalta et al., 2021). Decreasing isolation and building social networks increases life satisfaction in people managing all kinds of physical and psychological challenges (for a study that focuses on mental health in TGD communities, see Hall & Delaney, 2021). And a synthesis of the minority stress and TGD resilience literature makes several community-level recommendations for building reliance in TGD people, including social support, community belonging, and participating in activism (Matsuno & Israel, 2018).

DOI: 10.4324/9781003140740-13

There are several ways of thinking about community integration from a therapeutic standpoint. The first is through the lens of the therapy itself, in which the clinician becomes a member of the client's community, modeling secure, comfortable, and boundaried interpersonal relationships through the work of the therapy. The second is that a clinician can become a community *resource*, connecting a client to affirming spaces and activities, and acting as an accountability structure or sounding board to aid in the client's evaluation of how it feels to integrate or reintegrate with given or chosen family, or community based on shared interests or values.

THE THERAPIST AS COMMUNITY MEMBER

Virtually all therapeutic models encourage some type of integration or reintegration into the community, but both relational therapy and feminist therapy are intentional about centering the therapist-client relationship. Relational therapy operates explicitly from an attachment-based framework, with the intention of helping clients develop an internal working model of secure relationships (see Pearlman & Courtois, 2005, for a trauma-treatment focused overview). The clinicians describe four primary components of a strong therapeutic relationships, suggesting that the bond should be RICH by centering respect, information, connection, and hope. I like this relational model because it underscores the clinician's own development, rightly noting that for an attachment-based therapeutic relationship to be secure, the clinician must *also* be capable of secure relationships, including secure relationships with people who struggle to connect. Reliability, consistency, and pacing are discussed, and emotional availability and authenticity considered central. A more recent article asserts that all trauma therapy—and perhaps all therapy—is innately relational (Norcross & Wampold, 2019). These authors synthesize data regarding the import of the therapeutic relationship across studies centering a variety of trauma-treatment modalities. They go on to argue that it is the strength of the therapeutic relationship—as well as some factors of the relationship which are vested largely in the therapist—that has the strongest effect on treatment outcome. In terms of helpful implementation of therapeutic skills, they demonstrate that fitting the therapy to some aspects of the client's intersectional identity (they specify racial and ethnic culture and religious identity) and coping style will also improve efficacy. There is not specific relational work that I have seen which focuses on TGD people.

The theory of feminist therapy is rooted in the recognition that systemic inequality exists and has ongoing and significant impact on our lives and opportunities (Brown, 2018). Although it encourages the client to think about agentive action, they may be able to take to facilitate change in their life, it does so in dialogue with the recognition that structural barriers and facilitators have much greater power to define our lives and roles than individual choices. Feminist therapy focuses on agentive action in what it terms the four realms of power, which include the somatic, intrapersonal, interpersonal, and spiritual/existential. At least two of these realms, the interpersonal and the existential, center relationships, social context, and meaning-making. Although originally developed by and for white cisgender women, feminist therapy has expanded over time to incorporate a multiplicity of perspectives, and there is a forthcoming special edition of the journal *Women and Therapy* focused on feminist therapy clinical practice in TGD communities. This will include a perspective on feminist therapy with autistic TGD people (McConnell & Minshew, in press) as well as a discussion of the feminist therapy value of body acceptance as relates to gender incongruence (Joseph & Chavez, in press).

A treatment that is more in alignment with cognitive behavioral models of psychology, and yet centers the relationship between the clinician and client as a space for taking risks and trying out new relational possibilities, is acceptance and commitment therapy (ACT). ACT is a "third-wave" cognitive behavioral therapy that targets psychological rigidity in order to support clients in taking action in their own lives (see Hayes & Strosahl, 2005). In ACT, the therapist teaches the six core processes of the model; acceptance, diffusion, contact with the present moment, self as context, values, and committed action. The clinician then acts as a resource and guide for clients as they apply these skills for creating movement and change. For an overview of ACT as a treatment for PTSD and CPTSD, see McLean and Follette (2016). ACT has been adapted for many different client populations, and a recent article discusses adaptations (with clinical case examples) for use with TGD adolescents (Bennett & Dillman Taylor, 2019). For a model that fits data regarding psychological inflexibility to effects of gender minority stress, see Lloyd et al. (2019).

THE THERAPIST AS COMMUNITY RESOURCE

In Chapter 9, we discussed building a referral network of affirming health care providers, and I recommend you consider how this might extend to other areas of life. Look for peer support groups your TGD clients might be interested in attending, activist organizations they might get involved with, or opportunities to do art in affirming contexts. Engage with media by, for, and about TGD people, and be prepared to talk about TGD-centered media with your clients as well as other people in your life. Also take note when your clients tell you that an organization or institution is not living its values and be cautious about how/if you recommend it in the future.

Here are some specific questions you might ask as you try to gather resources for your TGD clients. This is by no means an exhaustive list:

- If one of your TGD clients has a rupture with their family of origin, do you know a support group for families of TGD individuals that could help heal that rift?
- Does your community have an LGBT+ center, and, if so, how is it regarded by TGD people?
- How are local organizations regarded by BIPOC feminine-spectrum people? Are there BIPOC feminine-spectrum people in positions of leadership there?
- How are local organizations regarded by fat people and disabled people? Is it accessible space? Are there low-stimulation offerings for autistic people? Chairs and sofas that are appropriate for fat bodies? ASL interpretation services?
- Does your area have affirming religious organizations? How are they regarded by TGD people? Can you build a relationship with the religious head of the institution?

HOW DOES THIS FIT WITH GENDER DEVELOPMENT?

In terms of the gender developments models of TGD gender development discussed in Chapter 8, all of these models agree that the social element of gender is a key component. Having our gender reflected by other people, cis and TGD, helps people see their gendered selves as real, valid, and worthy of care. When we see parts of ourselves as real, valid, and worthy of care, it becomes easier to feel that the terrible things that happened to us—although truly terrible and not to be dismissed lightly—were *part* of our experience, and we are not the entirety of who we are. When we are in community with people who have had similar gender trajectories, it becomes easier to believe in and trust our own gendered experiences.

FROM COMMUNITY INTEGRATION TO COMMUNITY CARE

More recently in my own development as a clinician, I have been thinking about the process of integration or reintegration into a community in a way that is less explicitly aligned with systems of psychotherapy, and more in alignment with what Schalk and Kim term feminist-of-color disability studies (2020). These theorists situate the sites of analysis for feminist-of-color disability studies in discourse, state violence, health/care, and activism. They also speak to the urgency of collective social mobilization toward disability justice. Disability justice does not center access to existing systems of power, but rather attends to the necessity of dismantling these oppressive systems and creating models that center the marginalized. There are many, many people more qualified to speak to this understanding of the importance of community and interdependence than I, whether you approach the topic from a perspective of fat justice (Harrison, 2021), disability justice (Piepzna-Samarashina, 2018), LGBT+ health (Sharman, 2021), or prison abolition (Kaba, 2021). An entry point for me was an essay that questions our understandings of the unspeakability of trauma (Spurgas, 2021). Is trauma really so unspeakable, this essay asks? Or do we struggle to hold it in community, thereby creating spaces that don't hear—or actively silence—the words of survivors? All of the above-mentioned authors center intersectional identity and speak to gendered experiences as mediated by systemic oppression and invisibilized structural trauma. If you are interested in thinking about these dynamics in your work with TGD people who have experienced stress and trauma, I encourage you to pick up these texts and see if there is anything in them that pushes against your worldview or leads you to question your treatment philosophy. For me, engaging with the ideas represented by these texts elicited a shift in my clinical frame. I used to think that community was important for my clients, and I still do. But what sometimes got lost in that formulation was the realization that communities also need my clients. We all need each other, in a stark and desperate way that is sometimes difficult and painful to recognize, but ultimately generative and fundamental to our humanity. As directly related to community integration, my takeaway is that TGD trauma survivors don't exactly benefit from being dependent on community, but rather we all benefit when we center *interdependence* and mutual care. As someone who was raised in a culture and class that clings to the myth of independence, this was a new way of thinking for me, and one with which I am still grappling.

BUILDING COMMUNITIES: THE CASE HISTORIES

Advika was primarily interested in maintaining and expanding relationships with members of their family of origin as their community, but in a way that felt true to their gender identity. She also really wanted accountability from her parents regarding their early bad reactions to her gender expression as a child. Advika struggled with feelings of guilt, fear, anger, and anguish as she worked toward this realization, and we redirected many times to in-session practices to build feelings of safety and security. They also began looking for dance classes and were ultimately able to find an instructor who gave private lessons online. Advika was never sure what this person believed about her gender identity, but ultimately she felt safe enough working with this instructor and excited enough to use her body in this way that she could tolerate her feelings of anxiety. Dance was further reinforcement for Advika that, while they were not a woman in the binary sense, they were certainly most comfortable on the feminine side of the gender spectrum.

Dance also provided an opportunity for Advika to talk with her mother about gender. They knew their mother would be happy to support dance lessons, as she had frequently expressed the wish that Advika resume dancing. But Advika did not want to try to pretend that she was studying dance forms for men. Advika's revelation about dance classes led to a longer and more involved conversation about their desire to start using estrogen. She was surprised by how openly her mother received this information and gratified by her mother's acknowledgment of her own hostile reaction to Advika's early expressions of gender fluidity.

Advika's father had a more difficult adjustment to Advika's coming out, and this had a chilling effect on their relationship. After a period of separation and reflection on all sides, however, he agreed that maintaining the familial relationship was important enough that he would work to reach toward Advika, although he did stipulate some conditions around his acceptance. This was a time in my relationship with Advika in which I had to be careful to check my impulses toward Western values of rugged individualism, and come to terms with the differences that can exist in very loving and connected families. Over time, it also reinforced for me the understanding that the first response to a coming out is not the last response, and that families really can grow together when everyone is invested and willing to offer the benefit of the doubt. Advika also benefited from advocacy on the part of one of her aunties, and has strengthened relationships with several cousins who supported her in the coming out process (including the cousin who unknowingly supplied her with her very first "girl clothes"). The strength of these relationships helped them through a period of disconnection with their father as well as exerted pressure on him to increase his acceptance of Advika's gender identity and expression.

Daniel found that he was most interested in reintegrating into a church community, but worried that he would not be able to find a church in which he felt valued and accepted. Fortunately, there is (at least) one predominantly Black and predominantly LGBT+ church in his city. (While I'm sure Daniel would have ultimately found his own way to this church, I had connected with the pastor through activism work in the past, and was able to tell Daniel about the church and reassure him that it would be a welcoming space for him.) He began attending Sunday services and then also a Bible study group for Black gay men. This eventually led to a romantic and sexual relationship with one of the other men. The relationship did trigger an increase in his alcohol use for a while, including a couple of pretty frightening incidents that encouraged him to step back from the relationship and do some reprocessing of childhood sexual trauma before re-engaging in the relationship. With the support of both his boyfriend and his pastor, he decided that he would like to do a medical detox from alcohol, but this became very complicated as the majority of inpatient programs are segregated by gender. Daniel had recovered from top surgery at this point, and his documentation all had M gender markers, but he was worried about ways that he might be outed if living with a group of other men without much privacy and also worried about the possibility of psychological or physical violence if this were to happen. Instead, he decided to work on tapering his alcohol use over time and ultimately joined a 12-step program in order to maintain his sobriety. This offered him another form of community connection, and the opportunity to provide mentorship (as a sponsor) to other gay men looking to maintain sobriety.

Shai had been very active in an online forum for disabled TGD people prior to the start of our work, and part of the circumstances that led them to me was an experience of being "called in" by the group for a series of abusive comments they had made in the group space. Shai was desperate to reunify with this group of people, I came to realize, but terrified of the accountability work that this would entail. We spent a great deal of time talking about rupture and repair as community processes, and they came to a place of recognizing their experience of this calling in as a parallel to being abandoned by, and ejected from, their family and religious community. As they came to trust our relationship, and the capacity to tolerate conflict that we had together, they slowly started to feel that perhaps the door with this community was not as closed as the door with their family of origin. They began approaching members of this forum and asking about making amends and the possibility of reunification. This was a slow and painstaking process. After all, Shai was not the only person in this community who had been rejected by their family of origin, or experienced significant trauma and maltreatment, and many people in the community held Shai as simply another abuser. There were definitely times where Shai became overwhelmed, swamped, and activated in making these approaches and also times in which Shai overwhelmed, swamped, and activated others. However, the sincerity of Shai's desire to change, and their commitment to the wellbeing of the community, provided a lot of motivation for moving forward even when it seemed impossible. This is currently an unfolding process, but Shai is in dialogue and in community with many members of this forum again and has been asked to be part of a working group for drafting community bylaws for navigating conflict in the community. Shai believes, and I agree, that this is part of the process of amends for them and is taking the process of drafting and iterating these bylaws very seriously.

IN SUM

In closing this chapter, and moving toward the end of this book, I'll state my fundamental beliefs about community in the simplest of terms. Community-building is not easy work, especially for people who have experienced trauma and stress. But it is necessary work, especially for people who have experienced trauma and stress. I hope you will remember this phase in working with TGD clients who have experienced trauma and stress.

WORKS CITED

Ainsworth, M. D. S. (1978). *Patterns of attachment: A psychological study of the strange situation.* Lawrence Erlbaum Associate.

Bennett, C. M., & Dillman Taylor, D. (2019). ACTing as yourself: Implementing acceptance and commitment therapy for transgender adolescents through a developmental lens. *Journal of Child and Adolescent Counseling, 5*(2), 146–160.

Bowlby, J. (1973). *Attachment and loss.* Hogarth Press and Institute of Psycho-Analysis.

Brown, L. S. (2018). *Feminist therapy* (2nd edition). American Psychological Association. https://doi.org/10.1037/0000092-000

Fern, J. (2020). *Polysecure: Attachment, trauma and consensual nonmonogamy.* Thorntree Press LLC.

Giovanardi, G., Vitelli, R., Maggiora Vergano, C., Fortunato, A., Chianura, L., Lingiardi, V., & Speranza, A. M. (2018). Attachment patterns and complex trauma in a sample of adults diagnosed with gender dysphoria. *Frontiers in Psychology, 9*, 60.

Hall, S. F., & DeLaney, M. J. (2021). A trauma-informed exploration of the mental health and community support experiences of transgender and gender-expansive adults. *Journal of Homosexuality, 68*(8), 1278–1297.

Harrison, D. L. (2021). *Belly of the beast: The politics of anti-fatness as anti-blackness.* North Atlantic Books.

Hayes, S. C., & Strosahl, K. D. (2005). *A practical guide to acceptance and commitment therapy.* Springer Science+ Business Media.

Joseph, J. A., & Chavez, J. R. (In press). Binding and queer embodiments: Rethinking the moral imperative of body positivity.

Kaba, M. (2021). *We do this' til we free us: Abolitionist organizing and transforming justice.* Haymarket Books.

Kozlowska, K., Chudleigh, C., McClure, G., Maguire, A. M., & Ambler, G. R. (2021). Attachment patterns in children and adolescents with gender dysphoria. *Frontiers in Psychology, 11*, 3620.

Lloyd, J., Chalklin, V., & Bond, F. W. (2019). Psychological processes underlying the impact of gender-related discrimination on psychological distress in transgender and gender nonconforming people. *Journal of Counseling Psychology, 66*(5), 550.

Main, M., & Solomon, J. (1986). "Discovery of a new, insecure-disorganized/disorientated attachment pattern. In M. W. Yogman & T. B. Brazelton (Eds.), *Affective development in infancy* (95–124). Ablex.

Matsuno, E., & Israel, T. (2018). Psychological interventions promoting resilience among transgender individuals: Transgender resilience intervention model (TRIM). *The Counseling Psychologist, 46*(5), 632–655.

McConnell, E. A., & Minshew, R. (In press). Feminist therapy at the intersection of gender diversity and neurodiversity.

McLean, C., & Follette, V. M. (2016). Acceptance and commitment therapy as a nonpathologizing intervention approach for survivors of trauma. *Journal of Trauma & Dissociation, 17*(2), 138–150.

Norcross, J. C., & Wampold, B. E. (2019). Relationships and responsiveness in the psychological treatment of trauma: The tragedy of the APA Clinical Practice Guideline. *Psychotherapy, 56*(3), 391.

Pearlman, L. A., & Courtois, C. A. (2005). Clinical applications of the attachment framework: Relational treatment of complex trauma. *Journal of Traumatic Stress, 18*(5), 449–459.

Piepzna-Samarasinha, L. L. (2018). *Care work: Dreaming disability justice.* Arsenal Pulp Press.

Porges, S. W., & Dana, D. (2018). *Clinical applications of the polyvagal theory: The emergence of polyvagal-informed therapies.* WW Norton & Company.

Schalk, S., & Kim, J. B. (2020). Integrating race, transforming feminist disability studies. *Signs: Journal of Women in Culture and Society, 46*(1), 31–55.

Sharma, S. R., Gonda, X., Dome, P., & Tarazi, F. I. (2020). What's love got to do with it: Role of oxytocin in trauma, attachment and resilience. *Pharmacology & Therapeutics, 214*, 107602.

Sharman, Z. (2021). *The care we dream of: Liberatory and transformative approaches to LGBTQ+ health.* Arsenal Pulp Press.

Sizemore, K. M., Talan, A., Gray, S., Forbes, N., Park, H. H., & Rendina, H. J. (2021). Attachment buffers against the association between childhood sexual abuse, depression, and substance use problems among transgender women: A moderated-mediation model. *Psychology & Sexuality.* https://doi.org/10.1080/19419899.2021.2019095

Spurgas, A. K. (2021). Solidarity in falling apart: Toward a crip, collectivist, and justice-seeking theory of feminine fracture. *Lateral, 10*(1), https://doi.org/10.25158/L10.1.9

Van Ijzendoorn, M. H., & Kroonenberg, P. M. (1988). Cross-cultural patterns of attachment: A meta-analysis of the strange situation. *Child Development, 59*(1),147–156.

Zalta, A. K., Tirone, V., Orlowska, D., Blais, R. K., Lofgreen, A., Klassen, B., ... Dent, A. L. (2021). Examining moderators of the relationship between social support and self-reported PTSD symptoms: A meta-analysis. *Psychological Bulletin, 147*(1), 33–54. https://doi.org/10.1037/bul0000316

CHAPTER 13

IN WHICH WE COME TO THE END OF OUR TIME TOGETHER

"Trans people don't have to weather the storm. We are the storm."

—Mara Keisling, then-Executive Director of National Center for
Transgender Equality, speaking on voting the president of
that epoch out of office, USPATH 2019

What an adventure this has been. The process of writing this book has helped me clarify my own values around gender-affirming care in the context of trauma treatment, and I hope it's a useful starting point in your own formulation of this work and what it means to you. In part, I hope it is helpful for you because gender-affirming treatment and therapy for trauma are both incredibly effective modalities that have the capacity to greatly improve the lives of our clients and community members.

For TGD people who are exploring identity, and for TGD children for whom medical interventions are not yet appropriate, participating in an uninhibited exploration of gender identity and expression can, if it is desired exploration, facilitate health and well-being. Over the years, a number of studies have indicated that TGD children struggle with psychopathology. This, however, is not intrinsic to the experience of gender diversity. TGD children who are supported in their identities endorse comparable levels of depression to cisgender children in their age cohort and only slightly elevated levels of anxiety (Olson et al., 2016). Among those TGD youth with a chosen name, using that name in school and home settings reduces negative health outcomes and mental health burden (Pollitt, 2021). While comparatively little is known about the health benefits of social transition exclusively for TGD adults, a recent review of the literature found that non-medical gender-affirmation (such as social transition and legal name change) was negatively associated with depression and other adverse mental health outcomes (King & Gamarel, 2021). Providing a nonjudgmental, exploratory space for people to talk and think about gender conceptually, *when people want this space*, has a beneficial psychological effect.

As discussed in previous chapters, gender-affirmative behavioral health treatment is sometimes also associated with gender-affirming medical interventions. For people who choose medical interventions, we know that hormone treatment decreases dysphoria and also can decrease experiences of depression and anxiety, in some cases eliminating the mental health disparity between TGD and cisgender people (Dhejne et al., 2016; Green et al., 2021). Indeed, a longitudinal study that found sub-threshold depression and anxiety in TGD individuals initiating hormone treatment found that self-reported depression and anxiety reduced over time after the initiation of hormone therapy (Colizzi et al., 2014). I'll reiterate here that psychological distress in TGD people is not an inevitability. When people of all genders are validated and supported in their genders, people of all genders can thrive (Hughto et al., 2020).

In addition to social transition and hormone transition, the data are clear for surgical transition: when people desire this treatment and are able to access it, their quality of life improves, and they are happier and more comfortable in the world. Secondary analysis of the 2015 USTS indicated that TGD people who had been able to access gender-affirming surgery endorsed less overall psychological distress, suicidality, and nicotine use in the year

DOI: 10.4324/9781003140740-14

prior to the survey than TGD people who had not been able to access these interventions (Almazan & Keuroghlian, 2021). Gender-affirming surgeries have satisfaction rates ranging from 94% to 100%, and regret is low (and usually centers on complications; van de Grift et al., 2018).

Trauma treatment improves life satisfaction as well. Having an understanding of how bodies and minds are impacted by trauma exposure, and an articulated vision for helping people move away from that impact is powerful. Whether someone engages in safety-focused approaches, approaches that center on reprocessing, or integration techniques, we have seen that there are bodies of literature that show that these trauma-informed treatments decrease symptoms of PTSD and increase quality of life and life satisfaction. While not every treatment works for every person, and improvement is not always easy to measure or quantify, people who get trauma treatment get better. Sometimes this means that people have fewer flashbacks and can manage the flashbacks they do have more effectively. Sometimes this means they are less impacted by dissociation, or generally happier, more connected, and more whole.

Therapy, then, can be helpful for our psyches and our minds. It can be helpful for our bodies and our brains. And, because we are social creatures embedded in social systems, what helps the individual has ripple effects for our community and our society. People who have resolved some of the difficulties of trauma exposure, or come to celebrate their TGD identity, or both, are better able to connect and contribute in community. When people are more comfortable in their bodies and minds, they are more available to relationships and have greater capacity to connect. To witness someone who has always believed that relationships are out of reach for them enter into a close friendship, intimate partnership, or healthy connection with a member of their family of origin is to witness a change in the fabric of someone's sense of self, and this is a change that indirectly benefits us all. When parents get the treatment they need, they can be more effective and available as parents, contributing to a cycle of intergenerational transmission of health and healing. When people get effective therapy, they are able to become better friends and more connected loved ones, in the sense that they will be able to communicate clearly, set boundaries, and live their full truth in a brave and open way.

In short, trauma-informed, gender-affirmative therapy works, but only if we practice it. In spending this time with me, Advika, Daniel, and Shai, you have learned some of the tools and information you need to be an integral part of this vital practice. Thank you for taking the time to engage with the joy, and the responsibility, of this vision. And now there is work to be done—in our bodies, our minds, and our communities.

What are we waiting for? Let's go!

WORKS CITED

Almazan, A. N., & Keuroghlian, A. S. (2021). Association between gender-affirming surgeries and mental health outcomes. *JAMA Surgery*, *156*(7), 611–618.

Colizzi, M., Costa, R., & Todarello, O. (2014). Transsexual patients' psychiatric comorbidity and positive effect of cross-sex hormonal treatment on mental health: Results from a longitudinal study. *Psychoneuroendocrinology*, *39*, 65–73.

Dhejne, C., Van Vlerken, R., Heylens, G., & Arcelus, J. (2016). Mental health and gender dysphoria: A review of the literature. *International Review of Psychiatry*, *28*(1), 44–57.

Green, A. E., DeChants, J. P., Price, M. N., & Davis, C. K. (2021). Association of gender-affirming hormone therapy with depression, thoughts of suicide, and attempted suicide among transgender and nonbinary youth. *Journal of Adolescent Health, 70*(4), 643–649.

Hughto, J. M., Gunn, H. A., Rood, B. A., & Pantalone, D. W. (2020). Social and medical gender affirmation experiences are inversely associated with mental health problems in a US non-probability sample of transgender adults. *Archives of Sexual Behavior, 49*(7), 2635.

King, W. M., & Gamarel, K. E. (2021). A scoping review examining social and legal gender affirmation and health among transgender populations. *Transgender Health, 6*(1), 5–22.

Olson, K. R., Durwood, L., DeMeules, M., & McLaughlin, K. A. (2016). Mental health of transgender children who are supported in their identities. *Pediatrics, 137*(3), e20153223.

Pollitt, A. M., Ioverno, S., Russell, S. T., Li, G., & Grossman, A. H. (2021). Predictors and mental health benefits of chosen name use among transgender youth. *Youth & Society, 53*(2), 320–341.

van de Grift, T. C., Elaut, E., Cerwenka, S. C., Cohen-Kettenis, P. T., & Kreukels, B. P. (2018). Surgical satisfaction, quality of life, and their association after gender-affirming surgery: A follow-up study. *Journal of Sex & Marital Therapy, 44*(2), 138–148.

INDEX

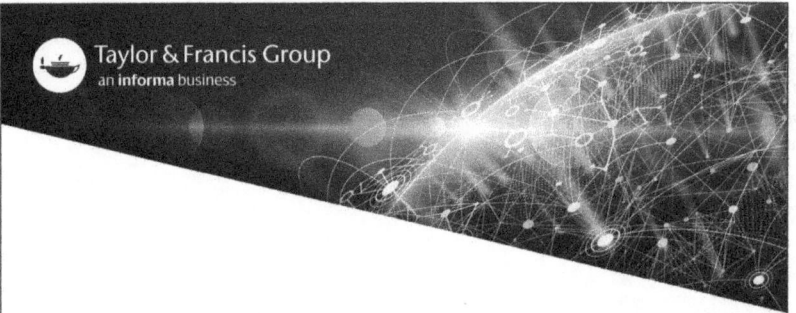
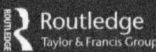
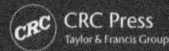